Evidence-based Practice for Nurses and Healthcare Professionals

4TH EDITION

Evidence-based Practice for Nurses and Healthcare Professionals

PAUL LINSLEY
ROS KANE
JANET BARKER

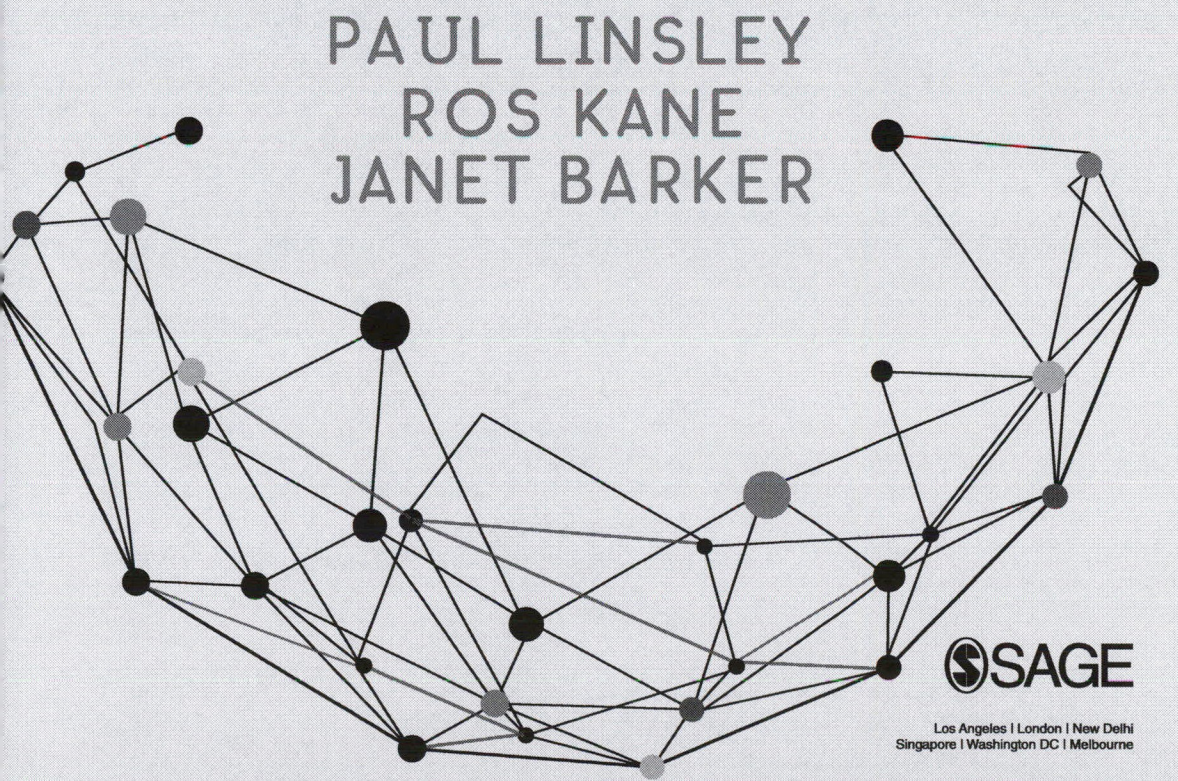

$SAGE

Los Angeles | London | New Delhi
Singapore | Washington DC | Melbourne

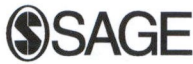

Los Angeles | London | New Delhi
Singapore | Washington DC | Melbourne

SAGE Publications Ltd
1 Oliver's Yard
55 City Road
London EC1Y 1SP

SAGE Publications Inc.
2455 Teller Road
Thousand Oaks, California 91320

SAGE Publications India Pvt Ltd
B 1/I 1 Mohan Cooperative Industrial Area
Mathura Road
New Delhi 110 044

SAGE Publications Asia-Pacific Pte Ltd
3 Church Street
#10-04 Samsung Hub
Singapore 049483

Editor: Alex Clabburn
Assistant Editor: Jade Grogan
Production editor: Tanya Szwarnowska
Copyeditor: Clare Weaver
Proofreader: Rosemary Campbell
Indexer: Martin Hargreaves
Marketing manager: Tamara Navaratnam
Cover design: Wendy Scott
Typeset by: C&M Digitals (P) Ltd, Chennai, India
Printed in the UK

First edition published 2009. Reprinted 2010, 2011 and
twice in 2012.
Second edition published 2013. Reprinted 2014.
Third edition published 2016. Reprinted 2017.
This fourth edition first published 2019.

Library of Congress Control Number: 2018957850

British Library Cataloguing in Publication data

A catalogue record for this book is available from
the British Library

ISBN 978-1-5264-5999-2
ISBN 978-1-5264-6000-4 (pbk)

At SAGE we take sustainability seriously. Most of our products are printed in the UK using responsibly sourced
papers and boards. When we print overseas we ensure sustainable papers are used as measured by the PREPS
grading system. We undertake an annual audit to monitor our sustainability.

Contents

About the Editors and Contributors

ABOUT THE EDITORS

Dr Paul Linsley has worked largely in acute and forensic mental health settings both as a clinician and as a manager. He sits on various national health and social care bodies and is an active researcher in his field of interest. Paul has presented at international conferences around the world and holds a wide range of awards. As a Senior Lecturer at the University of East Anglia he teaches on a number of courses, single and joint honours undergraduate programmes, research masters programmes and pre- and post-registration nurse training programmes in England. He has written on many mental health issues, including emotional intelligence, health informatics and the management of health care violence and aggression. He has an interest in values-based practice and engaging the service user as part of nurse education and this is reflected in this book.

Dr Ros Kane is a Reader in Healthcare and Director of Research in the School of Health and Social Care at the University of Lincoln in England. She co-leads the Mental Health, Health and Social Care Research Group (MH2aSC). With a background in nursing, Ros later graduated from University College London (UCL) with a BSc (Hons) in Anthropology and Geography and from The London School of Hygiene and Tropical Medicine (LSHTM) with an MSc in Medical Demography. Ros worked for ten years in the Centre for Sexual and Reproductive Health Research at LSHTM where she completed her PhD in 2005 (a study into the optimal provision of sexual health services for young people in England). She has a strong interest in quality improvement as well as service and policy evaluation, particularly in relation to sexual and reproductive health. Ros is a member of the Steering Group for the development of Clinical Academic Carers across the Midlands and East Region in England and is the lead for their clinical academic Bronze Scholar award, a pre-masters research programme for nurses, midwives and allied health professionals.

Dr Janet Barker has been involved in nursing for over 40 years, starting as a cadet nurse at 16 years of age in an orthopaedic hospital, moving into general nursing and finally working as a mental health nurse, in both inpatient and community settings. The last 20 years have been spent in nurse education. Janet has vast experience of organising and delivering undergraduate pre-registration nursing courses, taking on the role of Course Director of the Diploma/BSc (Hons) in Nursing programme at the University of Nottingham, School of Nursing, Midwifery and Physiotherapy in 2005. Janet received the University of Nottingham 'Dearing Award' in 2011 in recognition of her 'outstanding contribution to the development of teaching and student learning'. She retired as Associate Professor at the University of Nottingham in July 2011, however continues to keep abreast of current developments in nursing.

ABOUT THE CONTRIBUTORS

Dr Christine Jackson has a background in Radiotherapy and Oncology where she has worked in both clinical and academic environments. Her PhD relates to assessment of clinical competence in the newly qualified radiotherapy workforce. She has worked at the University of Nottingham in England as a multi-professional advisor for the Postgraduate Medical Deanery and the Trent Workforce Development Confederation. She has also worked in partnership with the Department of Health on a number of projects including the StLaR HR Project and the UKCRC subcommittee for nurses in Clinical Research. Christine was instrumental in working with Professor Tony Butterworth to establish the national framework for Clinical Academic Careers. She moved to the University of Lincoln in 2005 and led on the development of Clinical Academic Career Training. Christine is also a visiting professor at the University of Maribor in Slovenia and is co-founder and first chair of the international UDINE-C network (Understanding Development Issues in Nurse Educator Careers).

David Nelson is a Macmillan Research Fellow in the College of Social Science at the University of Lincoln in England, where he is a member of the Mental Health, Health and Social Care (MH2aSC) research group. His research aims to explore and compare the barriers and facilitators to self-management in people affected by cancer from rural and urban settings. In addition to research, David teaches quantitative and qualitative methods across the School of Health and Social Care on a range of undergraduate and postgraduate programmes. Prior to this, he worked in the School of Government and Public Policy at the University of Strathclyde and completed his BA (Hons) in Social Sciences at Glasgow Caledonian University and his MSc in Political Research at the University of Strathclyde. David is a member of the British Psychosocial Oncology Society (BPOS) and Social Research Association (SRA).

Marishona Ortega is a Chartered Librarian and has worked in the field of health and medical librarianship for twenty years both within the NHS and the academic sectors. Her professional interests include literature searching and evidence retrieval, systematic reviews and critical appraisal. She is a Fellow of the Higher Education Academy and is currently Senior Academic Subject Librarian: Bio-Medicine & Health Sciences at the University of Lincoln.

Amanda Thompson completed a BSc in Adult Nursing at Lincoln University in 2015. She is currently working as a staff nurse in the area of care of the older person. Prior to this she worked in the field of learning disabilities, primarily with young people with autism.

Publisher's Acknowledgements

The publishers are grateful to the following lecturers for their contribution to the book at review stage:

Thomas Beary, University of Hertfordshire

Petra Chipperfield, City University

Karen Heyward, University of Suffolk

Amelia Swift, University of Birmingham

Preface

Welcome to the fourth edition of *Evidence-Based Practice for Nurses and Healthcare Professionals.* The book is an essential resource for students and staff and highlights the importance of providing clinical practice based on sound evidence. It provides a clear and measured account of the increasing need for clinicians to be able to articulate the knowledge on which they make decisions and the part that evidence plays in driving practice forward. To practise effectively, nurses and other healthcare professionals need to be able to discern between the different sources of evidence available to them in order to make the best possible decisions in the interest of the patient at the time required. In order to do this, they need to be able to critically evaluate the evidence presented and make use of this in an informed way. This book explores the concept of evidence-based practice through a number of different lenses and provides practical guidance on its utilisation in clinical practice. The book has been revised to ensure that it remains contemporary and includes the provision of a new chapter on the history and development of clinical academic careers.

There are a number of ways in which this book can be used. Those new to the concept of evidence-based practice may want to work through the chapters chronologically to gain the necessary knowledge and skills in a step-by-step way. Those with some existing understanding may want use individual chapters as a point of reference, according to learning need. The book has also been written to support academic health and social care curricula and is a useful educational resource for a number of disciplines. Each chapter begins with a list of learning outcomes and ends with a summary of the main points, suggestions for further reading and useful weblinks. Key terms are highlighted, and definitions given in the glossary.

WHAT'S IN THE BOOK?

The book falls into three parts. Part I examines the key elements of evidence-based practice. Chapter 1 considers what EBP is and why it is important that practitioners understand and develop the necessary knowledge and skills to deliver it. Chapter 2 explores issues in relation to the nature of knowledge and where it comes from; what knowledge is seen as underpinning clinical practice; what counts as good and appropriate evidence. Chapter 3 highlights the important role that the public and patients play in developing new knowledge and moving practice forward. Chapter 4 considers issues related to clinical judgement, expertise and decision making. Chapter 5 discusses how to locate evidence and develop a search strategy and is very practical in its approach.

Part II provides an opportunity to explore the knowledge and skills associated with the critical appraisal of evidence, beginning with Chapter 6, which identifies what is meant by critical appraisal and its role in the EBP process. Chapters 7 and 8 look at critical appraisal specifically in relation to quantitative and qualitative research respectively. Chapter 9 considers issues related to systematic review and its place in evidence–based practice. Critical appraisal tools to help with this process are provided in the appendices.

Finally, Part III looks at how to make changes to practice once appropriate evidence has been identified and critically appraised. Chapter 10 discusses issues related to professional development, and how to ensure practice continues to be evidence based through the use of reflection and portfolio development. Chapter 11 considers how to integrate evidence into practice and how to begin to influence change generally and develop an evidence-based practice culture in the practice setting. Chapter 12 is a new chapter which examines the development of clinical academic careers and their impact on clinical practice and benefits for nurses, midwives and allied healthcare professionals.

The editors hope you will find the book a useful resource, one that helps you to develop the knowledge and skills needed to ensure patients receive the best care possible – based on good evidence and aimed at achieving positive outcomes.

PART I
Introducing Evidence-based Practice

1

Introduction: What is Evidence-based Practice?

Paul Linsley and Janet Barker

Learning Outcomes

By the end of the chapter you will be able to:

- define evidence-based practice;
- understand how evidence-based practice came into being;
- discuss the pros and cons of evidence-based practice;
- identify the components of evidence-based practice and the skills associated with it;
- consider why your practice needs to be evidence based.

INTRODUCTION

Evidence-based practice (EBP) is now a well-established concept on which the care and treatment of patients is based. Its introduction in the 1990s has had a direct impact on health and social care policy the world over and has led to, among other things, the expansion of the nurses' role. EBP is fundamental to the way in which nurses and other healthcare professionals approach their work, and in the decisions that they make. A nurse, like all other healthcare professionals, is primarily a knowledge worker. To practise effectively, healthcare professionals need to be able to discern between the different sources of knowledge available to them in order to make the best possible decision in the interests of the patient at the time required. For nurses, this translates into combining clinical evidence, individual expertise and patient preferences with the goal of providing good quality care. According to the Academy of Medical-Surgical Nurses (www.amsn.org/practice-resources/evidence –based–practice) the goals of EBP are:

- to give nurses the best evidence–based data available;
- to resolve problems in the clinical setting;
- to provide excellent care delivery;
- to reduce variations in care;
- to encourage effective nursing interventions;
- to help nurses make efficient and effective decisions in their work.

While there are a number of definitions defining EBP, perhaps the best known and accepted of these is that by Sackett et al. (1996) who defined EBP as:

> The conscientious, explicit, and judicious use of current best practice in making decisions about the care of individual patients. The practice of evidence-based medicine means integrating individual clinical experience with best available external clinical evidence from systematic research. (Sackett et al., 1996: 71)

This definition, while proving popular, has been criticised, as it seemingly ignores the contribution that patients play in the decision-making process. Muir Gray (1997) sought to address this shortfall in thinking by building on the work of Sackett and his team and put forward this definition of EBP in response:

> Evidence based practice is an approach to decision making in which the clinician uses the best evidence available, in consultation with the patient, to decide upon the option which suits the patient best. (Muir Gray, 1997: 3)

The above definition highlights the need to consult with the patient and involve them in decisions about their own health and wellbeing. It also takes into account patients' preferences, including their wish to avoid risks associated with interventions. Indeed, Sackett and his team (2000: 1) reviewed and developed a simpler but more telling definition of EBP in response to Gray's work, and defined EBP as:

> The integration of the best research evidence with clinical expertise and patient values.

This notion of patient involvement is echoed in more contemporary definitions of EBP, for instance:

> Evidence based practice entails making decisions about how to promote health or provide care by integrating the best available evidence with practitioner expertise and other resources, and with the characteristics, state, needs, values and preferences of those who will be affected. (Peile, 2004: 103)

EBP is more than using findings from research however. It is the integration of this **evidence** and knowledge into current clinical practice, for use at a local level, ensuring that patients receive the best quality care available. Implicit in such discussions is the message that healthcare, wherever it is delivered, must be based on good, sound evidence. It has been suggested that, historically, clinical issues have been based on a form of craft-based knowledge or 'habit, intuition and sometimes plain old guessing' (Gawande, 2003: 7). This is no longer sufficient and there is an expectation that strong evidence must underpin clinical practice. Indeed, healthcare professionals have a responsibility to practice evidence-based care, and this is reinforced in policy and guidance the world over.

> Reflect on the evidence that underpins your clinical practice. Where does this come from? How do you keep up to date with current developments and changes in practice? How easy is it to make changes to your practice using new evidence?

Activity 1.1

While the importance of research in the delivery of care has always been emphasised, the idea of evidence-based practice is seen as focusing the minds of those involved in care delivery on the use of appropriate evidence. Healthcare professionals need to be certain that their practice is current and up to date and that they are doing the best for those that they look after. EBP provides them with the means by which to explore practice and address any shortfall in the care that they give. The question then becomes one of how can the evidence be located? With the advent of the internet, busy healthcare professionals can no longer hope to keep up to date with all the possible sources of evidence, nor can they read and critically appraise all of the articles relevant to their practice. This is why an evidence-based approach to practice is needed. EBP provides a systematic framework for reviewing the evidence to underpin practice. There is a range of such evidence that can inform practice – personal experience and reflection literature, research, policy, guidelines, clinical expertise and audit (Dale, 2005) – all of which have their place within EBP and will be explored further in the various chapters of this book.

WHERE DID THE IDEA OF EBP COME FROM?

Professor Archie Cochrane, a British epidemiologist, is most frequently credited with starting the EBP movement. In his book *Effectiveness and Efficiency: Random Reflections on the Health Service* (Cochrane, 1972) he criticised the medical profession for not using appropriate evidence to guide and direct medical practice and challenged medicine to produce an evidence base. He argued there was a need to ensure treatment was delivered in the most effective manner and to ensure that available evidence was used in a consistent way.

When Cochrane talked of evidence, he meant randomised control trials (RCTs), which he viewed as providing the most reliable evidence on which to base medical care. RCTs are a form of research that use experimental designs to identify the effectiveness of interventions. The use of systematic reviews, which summarise the findings of a number of RCTs looking at similar areas of interest, was suggested as the 'gold standard' of the scientific evidence on which to base medical interventions.

The medical profession responded to Cochrane's challenge by creating the Cochrane Centre for systematic reviews, which opened in 1992 in Oxford. The Cochrane Collaboration was founded in 1993, consisting of international review groups (currently encompassing more than 28,000 people in over 100 countries) covering a range of clinical areas and producing systematic reviews. These reviews are published electronically, updated regularly and there are now over 4,600 available.

> **Activity 1.2**
>
> Visit the Cochrane Collaboration website (www.cochrane.org). How easy is the site to navigate? What sort of evidence does the site provide? How useful is the evidence? Could you readily relate/make use of this evidence as part of your clinical practice?

While the underpinning principles of evidence-based medicine (EBM) were hotly debated, the medical profession in general began to accept the idea, and 1995 saw the first issue of the journal *Evidence-Based Medicine for Primary Care and Internal Medicine*, published by the British Medical Journal Group. In 2007 EBM was identified as one of 15 major milestones in the development of medical practice since 1840 (*BMJ*, 2007). Nursing, emulating its medical counterpart, began to explore the notion of basing its practice on reliable sources of evidence, which resulted in the journal *Evidence-Based Nursing*, first published in 1998.

SOCIAL AND POLITICAL DRIVERS OF EBP

Scott and McSherry (2008) suggested a number of social and political factors facilitated the emergence of the emphasis on evidence at this time. The availability of 'knowledge' via the internet and other sources brought into being 'expert patients' – well-educated and informed individuals who accessed information relating to health and illness. Expectations of these expert patients were that healthcare professions would be aware of and use up to date information/research in their delivery of care and treatment. There was no longer a willingness simply to accept treatment or care purely on the advice of a doctor or nurse.

The concept of EBP was also seen as attractive by governments and health service administrators because of its potential to provide cost-effective and clinically effective care (McSherry et al., 2006). In the mid-1990s the UK government of the day identified that quality assurance was to be placed at the forefront of the NHS modernisation agenda. Two White Papers – *The New NHS: Modern and Dependable* (Department of Health [DH], 1997) and *A First Class Service: Quality in the New NHS* (DH, 1998) – outlined the plans for promoting **clinical effectiveness** and introducing **clinical governance**. These promoted systems to ensure quality improvement mechanisms were adopted at all levels of healthcare provision. Central to clinical governance were concepts of risk management and promoting clinical excellence. (See Figure 1.1 for an outline of the clinical governance framework).

Clinical effectiveness was defined by the NHS Executive (1996) as 'the extent to which specific clinical interventions when deployed in the field for a particular patient or population, do what they are intended to do, that is maintain and improve health and secure the greatest possible health gain'. This definition continued to underpin the more recent Department of Health approach to clinical effectiveness (DH, 2007a), with the various stages of the process being identified as:

- the development of best practice guidelines;
- the transfer of knowledge into practice through education, audit and practice development;
- the evaluation of the impact of guidelines through audit and patient feedback.

Put simply, clinical effectiveness can be seen as identifying appropriate evidence in the form of research, clinical guidelines, systematic reviews and national standards; changing practice to include this evidence; and evaluating the impact of any change and making the necessary adjustments through the use of clinical audit and patient feedback/service evaluation. Reading and understanding research, being aware of current policies and procedures, and knowing about the recommendations and standards in practice are all part of the nurse's role (Royal College of Nursing, 2007). Table 1.1 provides an overview of the key aspects of research, **clinical audit** and **service evaluation**.

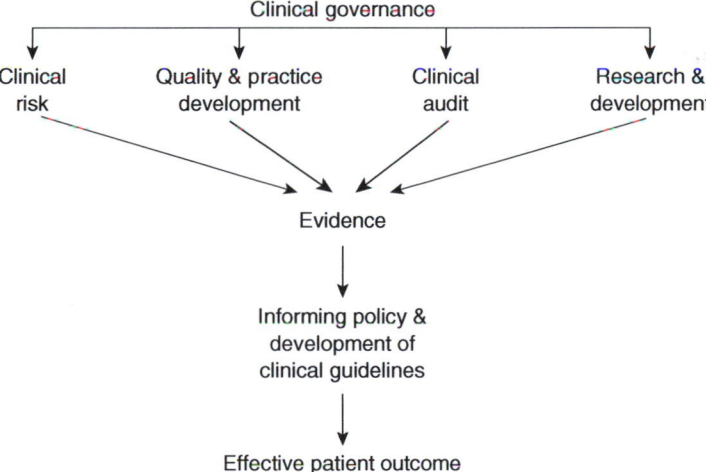

Figure 1.1 Representation of the elements of clinical governance

Two organisations were created aimed at promoting an evidence-based approach to healthcare, which are known today as the National Institute for Health and Care Excellence (NICE) and the Care Quality Commission (CQC). These bodies provide guidance for healthcare managers and practitioners and were charged with ensuring this guidance was followed in England and Wales. In Scotland the Health Technology Board fulfilled a similar purpose. Clinical governance was introduced to ensure healthcare was both efficient and effective; healthcare professionals were expected to show EBP supported all aspects of care delivery and service developments. It was hoped that the introduction of these measures would result in a shift in organisational culture from one that was reactive, responding as issues arise, to one with a proactive ethos, where the healthcare offered was known to be effective and, therefore, avoided unforeseen outcomes.

NICE and the CQC have continued to develop strategies to promote clinical effectiveness; the former through initiatives such as 'How to...' guides, quality standards and supporting a resource known as 'NHS Evidence'. The NHS Evidence site provides access to various forms of evidence that may be of use in clinical practice and provides examples of best practice. The CQC was charged with ensuring the safety and quality of care through inspection and assessment of all healthcare provision. The NHS Institute for Innovation and Improvement was set up in 2006 with a remit to support the implementation of service improvement initiatives within the NHS (although this was subsequently disolved).

Table 1.1   Research, audit and service evaluation

Research	Service evaluations*	Clinical audit
The attempt to derive generalisable new knowledge including studies that aim to generate hypotheses as well as studies that aim to test them	Designed and conducted solely to define or judge current care	Designed and conducted to produce information to inform delivery of best care
Quantitative research – designed to test a hypothesis. Qualitative research – identifies/explores themes following established methodologies	Designed to answer: 'What standard does this service achieve?'	Designed to answer: 'Does this service reach a predetermined standard?'
Addresses clearly defined questions, aims and objectives	Measures a current service without reference to a standard	Measures against a standard
Quantitative research – may involve evaluating or comparing interventions, particularly new ones Qualitative research – usually involves studying how intervention and relationships are experienced	Involves an intervention in use only. The choice of treatment is that of the clinician and patient according to guidance, professional standards and/or patient preferences	Involves an intervention in use only. The choice of treatment is that of the clinician and patient according to guidance, professional standards and/ or patient preferences

Research	Service evaluations*	Clinical audit
Usually involves collecting data that are additional to those for routine care but may include data collected routinely. May involve treatments, samples or investigations additional to routine care	Usually involves analysis of existing data but may include administration of interview or questionnaire	Usually involves analysis of existing data but may include administration of interview or questionnaire
Quantitative research – study design may involve allocating patients to intervention groups Qualitative research – uses a clearly defined sampling framework underpinned by conceptual or theoretical justifications	No allocation to intervention: the health professional and patient have chosen intervention before service evaluation	No allocation to intervention: the health professional and patient have chosen intervention before audit
May involve randomisation	No randomisation	No randomisation
Normally requires Research Ethics Committees (REC) review	Does not require REC review	Does not require REC review

*Service development and quality improvement may fall into this category.

Source: *Defining Research* (Health Research Authority, 2009).

> Identify one condition/disease you have come across recently in clinical practice. Visit the NICE website (www.nice.org.uk) and locate the NICE guidance and NHS evidence available in relation to your chosen condition/disease. Now ask the same questions you did of the Cochrane database: How easy is the site to navigate? What sort of evidence does the site provide? How useful is the evidence? Could you readily relate/make use of this evidence as part of your clinical practice?
>
> **Activity 1.3**

WHY DOES YOUR PRACTICE NEED TO BE EVIDENCE BASED?

The need for frontline staff to be empowered to deliver a quality service is a major aspect of contemporary healthcare policy. As Craig and Stevens (2011) have already identified, few would disagree with the ideas underpinning EBP – namely, that care should be of the highest standard and delivered in the most effective way. Indeed, practising without any 'evidence' to guide actions amounts to little more than providing care that is based on trial and error, which would not be advocated. However, as identified above, care is not always based on the best evidence, with Greenhalgh (2014) suggesting that many of the decisions made in healthcare are based on four main sources of information:

1. *Anecdotal information.* Here it is considered that 'it worked in situation X so it must be appropriate to (the similar) situation Y'. However, as Greenhalgh points out, while situations may seem very similar, patient responses are often very different.
2. *Press cuttings information.* Here changes are made to practice in response to reading one article or editorial, without critically appraising and considering the applicability of those results to the specific setting.
3. *Consensus statements.* Here a group of 'experts' will identify the best approaches based on their experiences/beliefs. While clinical expertise does have a place in EBP, it does not operate without some problems. For example, clinical wisdom once held (and to a certain extent still does hold) that bed rest was the most appropriate form of treatment for acute lower back pain. However, research in 1986 demonstrated that this is potentially harmful.
4. *Cost minimisation.* Here the limited resources available within a healthcare setting will often result in choosing the cheapest option in an effort to spread resources as widely as possible. However, EBP can ensure the most effective use of limited and pressurised resources. While certain types of care may appear more expensive on the surface, if these prove more effective, they may turn out to be cheaper in the long run.

Despite widespread recognition of the need for nursing practice to be based on sound evidence, frontline staff experience considerable challenges in implementing evidence-based care at an individual and organisational level. In particular, frontline nurses have difficulty interpreting research findings, and although willing to use research they often lack the skills to do so. Perhaps part of the problem related to nursing developing an EBP ethos is that it is often considered as more of an art than a science, and as such certain types of evidence are valued above others, such as expert opinion and practice experience. The complexities of healthcare, and the uncertainty of people's responses to and experiences of different types of interventions, require that full consideration is given to all available evidence.

Patients are likely to know a great deal about their own health needs and to expect health professionals to base care decisions on the most up to date and clinically relevant information. There is also an expectation that professionals will be able to comment in an informed way on any research reported in the media and identify its relevance to an individual's health needs. Miller and Forrest (2001) proposed that the ability to ensure that a professional's knowledge and skills remain current increases their professional credibility; allows them to be an important source of information to those in their care as well as colleagues; and enables all professionals involved in care delivery to make well-informed decisions. It has also been suggested that EBP can foster a lifelong learning approach – an essential requirement in the health professions if staff are to remain effective in rapidly changing healthcare environments (see Figure 1.2).

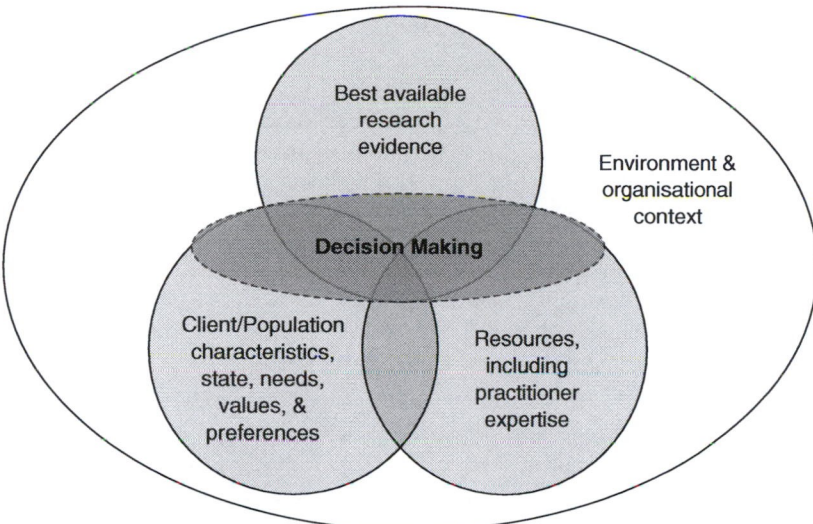

Figure 1.2 The integrated elements of EBP

Source: Council for Training in Evidence-Based Behavioral Practice (2008).

CONCERNS ABOUT EBP

Evidence-based approaches are not without their problems. As Wilkinson et al. (2011: 8) identified, it has both 'enthusiastic supporters and vociferous detractors'. Melnyk and Fineout-Overholt (2018) suggest that EBP is viewed by many as simply another term for research utilisation. It has also been argued elsewhere that the value of research has been over-emphasised to the detriment of clinical judgement and person-centred approaches, while others point to a lack of evidence to support the notion that EBP improves health outcomes.

Kitson (2002) has pointed to an inherent tension between EBP and person-centred approaches. She has argued that clinical expertise is vital in ensuring that patients' experiences and needs are not sidelined in the pursuit of 'best evidence' in the form of research findings and the development of generalised clinical guidelines. Some individuals have suggested that such broad general principles are not applicable to certain aspects of care. Wilkinson et al. (2011) suggested that practitioners often feel that an over-emphasis on EBP inhibits their ability to provide individualised care. Melnyk and Fineout-Overholt (2018) have identified this as a 'cookbook' approach, where a general recipe is followed with no consideration for the specific needs or preferences of individuals. There are concerns also around the ability to reach a consensus in relation to the various interpretations available when translating evidence into guidelines and the relevance of these for individual areas of practice. There are also issues related to the updating of evidence and the ability to ensure that the information gathered is current. However, DiCenso et al. (2008) argue that as clinical expertise and decision-making processes are central to EBP, in considering the use of general guidelines both of these processes must be used in the same way with any form of evidence including guidance.

Brady and Lewin (2007) argue that while the idea of clinical expertise is readily accepted by most experienced nurses, the majority of those same nurses are often unaware of the latest research in their area of practice. Nurses are generally presented as relying on intuition, tradition and local policies/procedures to guide their practice. There is also a perceived lack of enthusiasm in relation to the implementation of nursing research. Stevens (2013) proposed that healthcare providers frequently do not use current knowledge for a number of reasons, not least of these being the rapidly growing and changing body of research, some of which is difficult to apply to practice directly. As the aim of EBP is to deliver high-quality care, nurses need to have an understanding of what the exact elements of EBP are and to then develop the necessary skills and knowledge to enable them to carry this out. Glasziou and Haynes (2005) proposed that some research, essential to the delivery of quality care, will go unrecognised for years and suggested the major barriers to using evidence are time, effort and the skills involved in accessing information from the myriad of data available.

Ingersoll (2000) also argued that focusing EBP on care delivery reflects the differences between it and research. Research concentrates on knowledge discovery whereas in EBP the application of knowledge is central. In addition, she has suggested that while this emphasis on EBP is a welcome initiative, the wholesale 'lifting' of approaches and methodologies from another discipline such as medicine is not. Healthcare professionls need to make sure that the evidence used is relevant to their area of practice. There is a traditional view that evidence-based practice should be informed solely through quantitative research. However, Ellis (2010) advocates that it is more about using various forms of information, not just research, to guide and develop practice. Ellis (2010) goes on to note that there is little agreement between professionals as to what constitutes 'good evidence'. While nurses may be motivated to approach practice from an evidence-based perspective, the literature actually suggests that evidence-based practice is rigid and prescriptive, and diminishes any professional autonomy. French (1999) went further to suggest that as EBP is so closely linked with evidence-based medicine (EBM) and its preference for certain types of evidence, there is a danger that this promotes the use of medical knowledge over other forms and, therefore, leads to a medicalisation of healthcare environments to the detriment of other disciplines. Best evidence in the medical context is often taken to mean quantitative research findings in the form of RCTs. Some have questioned its compatibility with nursing and the other health professions, suggesting instead the use of a more open approach. Dale (2005) proposed that this issue has the potential to create interprofessional conflict, as that which nursing may count as appropriate evidence on which to base practice may be somewhat different from that of the medical profession.

Perhaps the biggest concern with EBP is that healthcare professionals may not have the necessary level of skill to interpret and make use of the evidence that they find. Advances in technology and scientific research possibilities and approaches further compound this. In addition, it is anticipated that there is little time allocated for learning these skills due to the busy and stressful nature of the profession. Healthcare professionals need both the knowledge and skills to make use of the available evidence that is both timely and worthwhile.

WHAT SKILLS ARE NEEDED?

While the idea for evidence-based medicine (EBM) grew out of Cochrane's work, McMaster Medical School in Canada is credited with coining the term in 1980 to describe a particular learning approach used in the school. This approach had four steps (Peile, 2004) and these are as follows:

1. Ask an answerable question.
2. Find the appropriate evidence.
3. Critically appraise that evidence.
4. Apply the evidence to the patient, giving consideration to the individual needs, presentation and context.

In addition to this, Aas and Alexanderson (2011) suggested a 'Five A' step process (see Figure 1.3). For the purposes of this book the authors have added an additional sixth stage, that of assess; this sits at the start of the cycle whereby the clinician identifies a problem and the need for further information and action. EBP should be all about doing – tackling real problems in clinical practice.

The most important element of the cycle is the asking of the question. The question should focus on the problem, the intervention and the outcome. Herbert et al. (2012) expanded the notion of the clinical question to include:

- effects of the intervention;
- patients' experiences;
- the course of the condition, or life–course (prognosis);
- the accuracy of diagnostic tests or assessments.

Evidence-based questions are usually articulated in terms of: What is the evidence for the effectiveness of x (the intervention) for y (the outcome) in a patient with z (the problem or diagnosis)?

Taking the above together, there is a need to develop particular skills and knowledge related to:

- the ability to identify what counts as appropriate evidence;
- forming a question to enable you to find evidence for consideration;
- developing a search strategy;
- finding the evidence;
- critically appraising the evidence;
- drawing on clinical expertise;
- issues concerned with patient preference;
- application to the context of care delivery;
- putting the evidence into practice.

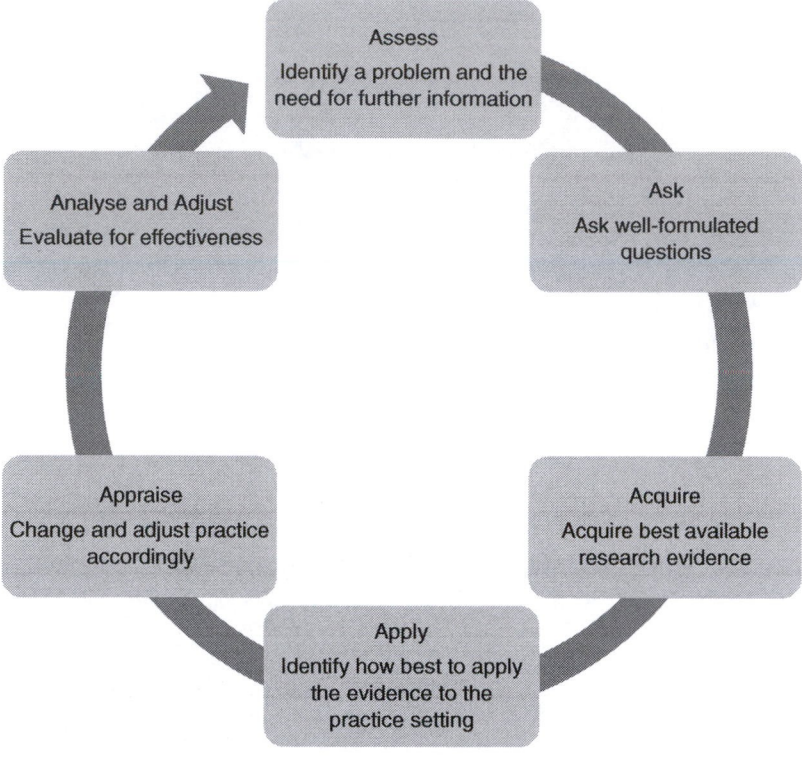

Figure 1.3   A 'Five A' plus one step approach to EBP

Activity 1.4

Consider the list of skills identified above as associated with EBP. Choose three areas that you feel you have most difficulty with and undertake a SWOT analysis in relation to each one using the grid in Appendix 1.

RESPONSIBILITY FOR EVIDENCE-BASED NURSING PRACTICE

The Canadian Nurses Association (2009) Position Statement on Evidence-Informed Decision-Making and Nursing Practice emphasises the role that not only nurses but other health professionals have in promoting and practising in an evidence-based way. These collaborative responsibilities go beyond the individual and extend to identifying and addressing barriers and enhancing factors within organisational structures and the health-care system that facilitate and promote evidence-informed practice. These responsibilities are as follows:

Individual nurses

- Are positioned to provide optimal care by having acquired competencies for evidence-informed nursing practice as part of their foundational education;
- Read and critique evidence-informed literature (i.e. research articles, reports) in nursing, health sciences and related disciplines;
- Generate researchable questions and communicate them to their manager or clinical nurse leaders or associated researchers;
- Participate in or conduct research; and
- Evaluate and promote evidence-informed nursing practice.

Professional and nursing specialty associations

- Use the best available evidence as a basis for standards and guidelines;
- Lobby governments for funding to support nursing research and health information systems that include nursing care data;
- Lobby governments for healthy public policy, regulation and legislation that are evidence-informed.

Researchers

- Identify knowledge gaps and establish research priorities in conjunction with clinicians and/or other health professionals, key stakeholders and client groups;
- Generate high-quality evidence through research;
- Facilitate capacity building of new nurse researchers; and
- Engage in effective knowledge transfer, translation and exchange to communicate relevant findings of the results of research to those who require the information.

Educators and educational institutions

- Support those graduating from basic and continuing nursing education programmes to acquire competencies to provide evidence-informed nursing;
- Use and develop evidence-informed curricula by providing high-quality education in research methods, evidence collection and analysis; and
- Promote a spirit of inquiry, critical thinking, openness to change and a philosophy of life-long learning.

Health service delivery organisations

- Reduce barriers against and enhance the factors within organisations that promote evidence-informed practice by intergrating research findings and practice guidelines:
- Evaluate outcome measures through ongoing audits and formal research studies;

- Support registered nurses' involvement in research and in the transfer of research into organizational policy and practice; and
- Provide continuing education to assist nurses to maintain and increase their competence with respect to evidnce-informed practice.

Governments

- Support development of health information systems that support evidence-informed nursing practice;
- Support health information institutions; and
- Provide adequate funding to support nursing research in all its phases.

Source: Canadian Nurses Association (2009) *Position Statement: Evidence-Informed Decision-Making and Nursing Practice*. Ottawa. Adapted with permission.

The list emphasises the prominent role that nurses, and clinicians, have to play in promoting evidence-based practice. From ensuring that their practice is up to date and based on the best evidence available, to adding their voice and weight to local and government initiatives, as well as playing an active part in and initiating research studies of their own. It also emphasises the importance of communication between groups and the need to disseminate and make use of best evidence to inform care and service provision. These topics and processes will now be explored in greater depth in the chapters that follow.

Summary

- EBP is a global phenomenon that promotes the idea of best practice, clinical effectiveness and quality care and involves an integration of evidence, clinical expertise, patient preferences and the clinical context of care delivery to inform clinical decision making.
- EBP focuses on critically appraising evidence to support care delivery rather than on research to discover new knowledge.
- The emergence of the expert patient has given rise to the need for health professionals to ensure they are up to date and their care is based on the best evidence available.
- Government initiatives have promoted EBP as a way of providing both clinically effective and cost-effective healthcare.
- Various steps are associated with the EBP process – forming a question; finding evidence; critically appraising the evidence; integration of evidence into practice.
- The knowledge and skills associated with EBP are an essential component of nursing practice.

FURTHER READING

Greenhalgh, T. (2014) *How to Read a Paper: The Basics of Evidence-Based Medicine* (5th edn). Oxford: Wiley-Blackwell/BMJ Books.

Rycroft-Malone, J., Seers, K., Titchen, A., Harvey, G., Kitson, A. and McCormack, B. (2004) 'What counts as evidence in evidence-based practice?', *Journal of Advanced Nursing, 47*(1): 81–90. This article gives a clear overview of the evidence-based movement and issues related to the nature of evidence.

Spruce, L. (2015) 'Back to basics: implementing evidence-based practice', *AORN Journal,* Jan *101*(1): 106–12.

USEFUL WEBLINKS

Cochrane Collaboration: promotes, supports and prepares systematic reviews, mainly in relation to effectiveness. www.cochrane.org

Joanna Briggs Institute: promotes evidence-based healthcare through systematic reviews and a range of resources aimed at promoting evidence synthesis, transfer and utilisation. www.joanna briggs.org

National Institute for Health and Care Excellence: provides guidance and other products to enable and support health professionals deliver evidence-based care. www.nice.org.uk

2

The Nature of Knowledge, Evidence and How to Ask the Right Questions

Ros Kane, Janet Barker and Amanda Thompson

Learning Outcomes

By the end of the chapter you will be able to:

- discuss the nature of knowledge;
- identify what is meant by 'evidence';
- form a question to allow identification of best evidence;
- understand the use of the PICO framework in forming research questions;
- understand how values-based practice complements evidence-based practice;
- demonstrate awareness of the principles of research ethics and governance.

INTRODUCTION

Knowledge is defined as: 'Facts, information, and skills acquired through experience or education; the theoretical or practical understanding of a subject' (*Oxford English Dictionary*, 2018). It is suggested that humans have a basic need for knowledge and a thirst to know how things work and why things happen. Parahoo (2014) proposed that knowledge is essential for human survival, and central to decision making about daily life and achieving change in both people and the environment in which they live. Prior to the eighteenth century much of people's understanding of the world and how it worked was based on beliefs related to superstitions and organised religions. However, the eighteenth century ushered in what we know as the era of 'Enlightenment' and the 'Age of Reason' which promoted different ways of thinking and knowing the world. The work of encyclopaedists (generally the leading philosophers of the day) and the publication of the *Encyclopedie* in the period from 1751 to 1772 together advocated scientific knowledge. This type of knowledge influenced thinking about the nature of humans and their ways of understanding the world, and from this came an opening of the debate about what knowledge is and how humans can 'know' things.

Knowledge and evidence are inextricably linked – evidence provides support to the usefulness of certain types of knowledge and knowledge gives reason and value to different forms of evidence. Therefore, as with knowledge, there are many different forms of evidence, each of which will be valued in different ways according to context.

This chapter will consider the issues surrounding the nature of knowledge, the different forms of evidence and how it is possible to identify what knowledge is needed to ensure practice is evidence based.

NATURE OF KNOWLEDGE

Knowledge is broadly categorised into two types – **propositional** and **non-propositional**. Propositional or codified knowledge is said to be public knowledge, and is often given a formal status by its inclusion in educational programmes. Non-propositional knowledge is personal knowledge linked to experience, and is described by Eraut (2000) as a 'cognitive resource' – a way of making sense of things – that someone brings to any given situation to help them think and act. It is often linked to '**tacit**' **knowledge**. This is knowledge that often difficult to put into words. For instance, people may know how to ride a bike and know how they learnt to do it, but may not be able to describe critical aspects, such as how they keep their balance. In considering where knowledge comes from Kerlinger (1999) identified three sources – **tenacity**, **authority** and **a priori**. Tenacity relates to knowledge that is believed simply because it has always been held as the truth. Authority relates to knowledge that comes from a source or person viewed as being authoritative and, therefore, must be true. A priori knowing relates to reasoning processes, where it is reasonable to consider something to be true. It is suggested that all three sources of knowledge are viewed as being objective in nature and not based on a person's subjective view of the world (see Box 2.1 for examples of these types of knowledge).

Box 2.1 Examples of three sources of knowledge

An individual with a cold knows that taking cough mixture will soothe their cough. If asked how they know this they might answer:

- 'because I know it does' – tenacity;
- 'because my mother told me it does' – authority;
- 'because it stands to reason that cough medicine will soothe a cough' – a priori.

It has been suggested that in relation to clinical decision making there are four forms of knowledge available to practitioners – superstition, folklore, craft and science (Justice, 2010). Superstition is similar to tenacity in that it is a belief that has no rational basis, such as the belief that bad things always happen in threes. Folklore relates more to a pattern of beliefs put forward at an earlier time, which are slow to be replaced by other, more feasible explanations for behaviours, such as the belief that the cycles of the moon affect the behaviour of people with mental health problems. Craft-based knowledge is seen most commonly as being practice-based knowledge – gained through clinical experience and drawing on personal judgement and intuition. However, there may well be a theoretical aspect, often gained during initial professional education. Science is a broad term relating to the ways of understanding the world. It is frequently thought to have a uniform definition; however, as will be discussed below, there are different views as to what can be deemed 'scientific knowledge'.

Activity 2.1	Think about recent experiences in practice. Can you identify examples of knowledge that are based on tenacity, authority and a priori sources, and also those that appear to have their basis in superstition, folklore and craft knowledge?

PHILOSOPHICAL UNDERPINNINGS OF KNOWLEDGE AND RESEARCH

The term **science** comes from the Latin word *scientia*, meaning knowledge. Such knowledge has traditionally been seen as being based on observation, experiment and measurement (Mason and Whitehead, 2011). Scientific knowledge is usually generated either through **deductive** or **inductive reasoning** (Streubert and Carpenter, 2010). Deductive reasoning is said to move from the general to the particular, while inductive reasoning moves from the particular to the general. With deductive reasoning a researcher would start with a hypothesis, which she or he would then seek to prove. A **hypothesis** is a simple statement that identifies a cause and effect relationship between two things – if I do X then Y is likely to happen. For example, in relation to considering the use of wound dressings (the general issue) a nurse might consider that one form of dressing (the particular) is more effective than another. The hypothesis might be that wound dressing A will promote more rapid wound healing than dressing B. In inductive reasoning, a nurse might start by considering somebody's experience of leg ulcers (a specific issue); she or he could then interview various people who have the condition, asking them about their experiences. Once a number of views have been collected it is possible to draw conclusions and a general theory of the experience could then be developed.

Ontology – the study of reality and how it can be understood (Ormston et al., 2014) – has evolved to encompass a range of theoretical positions on the nature of social reality and modes of apprehension: **realism** posits that there exists an external reality independent of subjective human perceptions; **materialism** (a variant of realism) proposes that reality is only perceptible through material features such as economics; while the position of **idealism** holds that reality can only be apprehended through the mind which constructs meaning or attaches it to experience.

Deductive reasoning is often associated with **positivism**, the idea that reality is ordered, regular, can be studied objectively and quantified. A basic component of positivism is **empiricism**, where it is proposed that only that which can be observed can be called fact or truth. This positivist or empirical way of looking at the world is based on a belief that 'reality' is external to and independent from humans but that humans can, by objectively observing the world around them, uncover knowledge that is true. Originally, such observation was intended to mean observation by human senses – sight, touch and so on. However, over time this has been expanded to include indirect observation through the use of specific tools designed to help a scientist observe and record phenomena. So, whereas the study of personality could be viewed as impossible because it cannot be seen, the development of a personality inventory provides a tool that the scientist can use to study it empirically. The idea of 'cause and effect' is also important in empiricism – if I do this (cause) then this (effect) will happen – so, for example, if dressing X is used (cause) the wound will heal more quickly (effect). Empiricism is often described as reductionist, which relates to the breaking down of areas of interest into small parts rather than considering the whole.

The positivist way of looking at the world developed particularly from scientific methods used in maths and physics and emphasises the need for objective and unbiased enquiry. The positivist worldview came to dominate scientific enquiry into the natural world. The more recent development of scientific enquiry into the social world (the social sciences include psychology, sociology and anthropology – these subjects explore how human beings think, behave and interact with each other and with their environment) found the positivist worldview to be limited in generating knowledge about the social world. **Interpretivism** – a different worldview – emerged from the social sciences.

Inductive reasoning is linked with interpretivism, an alternative to positivism based on the belief that humans are actively involved in constructing their understanding of the world. It is proposed that individuals constantly strive to understand what is happening in their environment and interpret action and interaction in an effort to make sense of their experiences. From this perspective, it is proposed that there is a range of views of the world and ways of understanding, depending on the interpretation people give to their experiences. Rather than adopting reductionist approaches and identifying cause and effect, interpretivism is seen as considering the whole, exploring all the subjective values and meanings that people attach to their experiences and seeking a full as possible understanding of phenomena. The interpretivist understanding is not arrived at objectively by 'pure' observation (as is the aim of the positivist worldview) but is approached inductively by exploring subjective experience. The role of the researcher using an interpretivist approach has to be acknowledged as another layer of interpretation – that is, in the process of interpreting their findings they may be influenced by their own values and experiences (Ormston et al., 2014).

As can be seen from the above, philosophical positions are adopted about the nature of the world, what can be known and how to gather this knowledge. These philosophical positions are known as **paradigms**, a term first created by Kuhn (1970). A paradigm is a set of logically connected ideas which guide the way in which research can be conducted – the methods used, the form of data collected and how that data are analysed. These design aspects of research must clearly support the uncovering of knowledge that will be perceived as having truth value. Two paradigms are generally accepted as being present in research – qualitative and quantitative – based on two different and sometimes competing ways of discovering the world. Researchers must consider carefully which paradigm or worldview best fits with the knowledge they are seeking to uncover – the design of their research must align with its purpose (LoBiondo-Wood and Haber, 2017). Qualitative research is concerned with exploring the meanings people attach to experiences and generating theories, whereas quantitative research is focused on generating data to prove or disprove theories. The paradigms are reflected in the way data are collected: put simply, qualitative data tend to be in the form of words, what people say about their experiences; quantitative data are presented in the form of numbers providing a basis for statistical analysis. Examples of how research into the same general area might look are given in Table 2.1.

Table 2.1   Examples of research questions

An investigation of anxiety in patients	
What is the nature of anxiety in patients? What sorts of things provoke anxiety and what is the relationship between them?	Are patients who are supplied with information less anxious than those who are not?
This is a qualitative approach ... the question is a 'what IS this?' type. Suggests an inductive approach, moving from the specific to the general.	This requires a quantitative approach. Suggests a cause and effect relationship and then tests it.

Table 2.2   Differences between quantitative and qualitative research

Quantitative	**Qualitative**
Scientific principles	Understanding/meaning of events
Moves from theory to data	Moves from data to theory
Identification of causal relationships between data	A close understanding of the research context
Collection of adequate amount of data	Collection of 'rich/deep' data
Application of controls to ensure validity	Seeks to address all aspects of the issues
Highly structured	Flexible structure allowing for changes in emphasis
Objectivity	Researcher as part of the process
Acceptance/rejection of hypothesis/laws	Generation of theory

Quantitative methods include randomised control trials (RCTs), experimental designs and involve statistical analysis of data. Qualitative enquiry includes phenomenology, ethnography, action research and grounded theory and generally involves interviews and observation, although some forms may incorporate aspects of statistical analysis. Table 2.2 provides a brief summary of the differences between qualitative and quantitative approaches. Issues related to the research approaches are discussed in further detail in Chapters 7 and 8.

AN EXAMPLE FROM NURSING

There is much debate as to what constitutes nursing knowledge. Knowledge plays a complex role in professions, often being seen as a defining trait. Schön (1990) suggested there is a hierarchy of knowledge in professions:

- basic science;
- applied science;
- technical skills of everyday practice.

He also suggested that professions' status is dependent on this hierarchy, that the closer a professional knowledge base is to basic science the higher the status. Nursing has tried for many years to establish a defined scientific knowledge base. Huntington and Gilmour (2001) stated that nursing has traditionally focused on empirical approaches to knowledge generation and has used these to explain the nature of nursing practice. The development of this knowledge has been influenced by other disciplines such as medicine, psychology and sociology. Although for a number of years scientific knowledge has been accepted as superior to other forms, more recently this has been challenged and there is a growing belief that other forms of knowledge are essential in the practice of nursing.

Carper (1978) was one of the first people to provide a framework through which the patterns of knowing in nursing could be considered. She identified four types of nursing knowledge – empirical, personal, aesthetic and ethical – and suggested that no one form of knowledge is superior to another; instead, each was essential to the practice of nursing. Empirical knowledge is the theoretical and research-based knowledge that is generated through systematic investigation and observation. This may also be knowledge generated by other disciplines, which can be seen as either a theory underpinning practice (such as anatomy and physiology) or a theory translated for use in nursing in a unique way (as with applied sciences such as psychology). Chinn and Kramer (2018) added the development of nursing theory to the concept of empirical knowledge, particularly in relation to interpretive research approaches such as phenomenology.

Personal knowledge relates to the individual nurse's experience of the world generally and nursing specifically. It encompasses that person's beliefs, values, perception and level of self-awareness. In many ways it resembles reflective practice, as implicit within this is the ability to know oneself and how this influences one's practice. The emotional aspects of nursing require nurses to consider how and why they respond to certain situations in certain ways to ensure the care they deliver is appropriate and compassionate. This type of knowledge is something that is seen as changing over time and having direct implications on the type and form of interactions that occur between nurses and patients.

Aesthetic knowledge is described as that knowledge which underpins the 'art' of nursing and health care. It can be seen as a bringing together of the manual, technical and intellectual skills aspects of nursing, particularly in nurse and patient interactions. This type of knowledge is often linked to expert practice and the ability to assist individuals in coping with health issues in a positive way.

Finally, ethical knowledge is seen as focusing on what is right, appropriate and moral; it relates to the judgements to be made in relation to nursing actions. It is also related to codes of conduct, procedural guidelines and the philosophical principles that underpin nursing.

Activity 2.2

Reflect on a recent clinical placement. Can you identify specific incidents where you used Carper's four types of knowledge?

Table 2.3 gives examples of activities associated with the different types of knowledge identified by Carper.

Intuition is an area that has been the subject of much debate, with what is termed **intuitive knowledge** being seen by many as an important aspect of clinical practice. Intuition can be defined as the 'instant understanding of knowledge without evidence of sensible thought' (Billay et al., 2007: 147) and is often considered to be a form of tacit knowledge. It is the moment when someone 'knows' that something is going to happen, or reaches a conclusion, without being aware of thinking in a rational and logical way to arrive at that point.

Table 2.3   Examples of activities associated with different types of knowledge

Knowledge	Example
Empirical	Biological sciences knowledge to understand blood pressure readings
	Psychology theory in relation to phobias to understand a patient's fear of injections/needles
Personal	'Therapeutic use of self' in understanding a person's response when given 'bad news'
	Interpersonal relationships, therapeutic relationships
Ethical	Code of conduct
	Confidentiality

Knowledge	Example
Aesthetic	Communicating with a patient in a caring and appropriate way before giving an injection
	Recognising the individual needs of a person when helping them with personal hygiene

In considering the nature of intuition in professional practice, Benner (1984) suggested that a form of practice knowledge or 'expertise' exists which is part of expert practice. Here, healthcare professionals draw on all their empirical and personal knowledge to reach a conclusion, without being aware of processing the information (see Box 2.2 for an example). Benner differentiates between practical and theoretical knowledge, suggesting that the former relates to 'knowing how' and is related to skills and the latter to 'knowing that', which is concerned with the generation of theory and scientific knowledge. However, she also suggested that in nursing, as expertise develops, a form of practice knowledge is apparent that 'side steps' the logical reasoning processes associated with science. Extending the knowing how through practice experience can lead to knowledge that appears to be available to the person without the aid of analytical process but which nevertheless is valid.

Box 2.2   Example of expert knowledge (Benner, 1984: 32)

An extract from an interview with a nurse who worked in the psychiatric setting for 15 years:

> When I say to a doctor 'this patient is psychotic', I don't always know how to legitimise that statement. But I am never wrong. Because I know psychosis from inside out. And I feel that, and I know it, and I trust it. I don't care if nothing else is happening, I still really know that. It's like the feeling another nurse described in the small group interview today, when she said about the patient 'she just isn't right'.

Other forms of knowing have been added to Carper's original work. For example, Mullhall (1993) put forward the idea of 'unknowing', proposing that nurses needed to make deliberate attempts to be open to new ideas and ways of thinking; seeing this as a step in building knowledge and a deeper understanding of individual practice experiences. Socio–political knowledge was included by White (1995). Here, political awareness, cultural diversity and public health agendas are essential aspects of knowing, enabling nursing to see its practice in a broader arena. Chinn and Kramer (2018) proposed 'emancipatory knowledge', that is, an awareness of social inequalities and their implication for health, including a political awareness, the need for social change and methods to bring this about.

WHAT CONSTITUTES EVIDENCE?

The dictionary definition of evidence is 'The available body of facts or information indicating whether a belief or proposition is true or valid' (*Oxford English Dictionary*, 2018). Pearson (2005) proposed in healthcare that it is 'data or information used to decide whether or not a claim or view should be trusted'. What exactly constitutes evidence in EBP is still hotly debated. Thomas (2004) suggested that evidence is information that is seen as relevant to how to provide care and beliefs about health and illness. Various hierarchies of evidence have been generated which clearly place quantitative findings from systematic reviews of RCTs at the top of the hierarchy; often qualitative research findings are not included within these hierarchies at all (see Chapter 5 for a more detailed discussion of evidence hierarchies). This preference for one form of evidence over another perhaps comes from the Cochrane Collaboration, which focused on the effectiveness of interventions for which RCTs are ideally suited and also on the dominance of the positivist paradigm in terms of research approaches. However, there is a growing body of literature that hotly contests the placing of RCT methods at the top of the hierarchy. Scott and McSherry (2008) suggested that RCTs are not always the most pertinent approach to certain aspects of nursing care. As discussed above, different ways of exploring the natural and the social worlds have developed and the practice of nursing encompasses both natural and social sciences.

Porter and O'Halloran (2012) assert that RCTs do not provide the best evidence for the complex systems in which healthcare is delivered. Different types of research questions require different forms of study. Therefore, the most appropriate form of evidence is that which relates to the question being asked – 'horses for courses' as Petticrew and Roberts (2003) put it.

Nursing has long recognised that its practice is based on multiple ways of knowing, and much of nursing activity does not fit easily with an RCT approach. The advocating of one type of evidence as superior to another is not helpful in providing evidence on which to base practice in a profession as multifaceted and complex as nursing. It is suggested that perhaps it is more appropriate to acknowledge the possibility of multiple hierarchies, depending on the object or issue under consideration. Nairn (2012: 14) proposed 'there is one world, but multiple ways of examining that world'.

The Joanna Briggs Institute (JBI) supports the idea of there being a range of issues that need to be considered in healthcare, and that different forms of evidence are needed. It is suggested that evidence generally falls into four areas:

1. Evidence of feasibility – whether something is practical/practicable physically, culturally or financially. In this situation one type of treatment might be the most effective, but financially unaffordable. For example, the cost of certain drugs means they are not used in certain healthcare systems. Types of evidence to support this would probably be economic and policy research.
2. Evidence of appropriateness – whether a particular intervention fits with the context in which it is to be given. For example, blood transfusion within certain religious groups might not be an appropriate form of treatment. Research considering ethical and philosophical issues would be of use here.

3. Evidence of meaningfulness – how interventions/activities are experienced by individuals. For example, the patients' experiences of or beliefs about fertility treatment might influence how services are organised. Interpretive research in the form of phenomenology, ethnology or grounded theory would be of interest in this area.
4. Evidence of effectiveness – whether one treatment is better than another or the usual intervention. RCTs and cohort studies would be of use here.

Rycroft-Malone et al. (2004a) suggested four types of evidence on which nurses can base their practice:

1. Research.
2. Clinical experience.
3. Service user/carer perspectives.
4. Local context.

They went on to identify that the challenge is in knowing how to integrate these four types of evidence in a robust and patient-centred way.

Ensuring the robustness of evidence related to clinical experience requires the gathering and documenting of this experience in a systematic manner, allowing for individual and group reflection and cross-checking. Portfolios and clinical supervision are methods which can enhance the validity of this type of evidence and these are explored further in Chapter 11. A crucial skill for nurses to develop is the ability to scrutinise and critically evaluate the quality of evidence. Chapter 6 introduces a number of research tools which help to develop these skills and can be of use in practice.

THE ROLE OF VALUES

Recent scrutiny of the NHS in the UK has led to a recognition of the need to reflect on current culture and practice and the revisiting of the values which underpin practice (McGonagle et al., 2015). In England, the Department of Health (DH) has set out a commitment to values in the NHS constitution (DH, 2013). Central to this is the understanding that patients are at the core of decision making, not simply passive recipients of care or treatment.

Values-based practice (VBP) is an approach to healthcare delivery that seeks to complement evidence-based practice (EBP) (Fulford, 2008). It is the utilisation of skills to promote balanced decision making in patient care, while also accounting for the complex web of differing value perspectives which lie behind the decision-making process. Much has been written about the place of VBP in the delivery of care (Fulford et al., 2012). It is predicated on the belief that different perspectives need to be respected, especially when dealing with challenging topics. The respect for alternative points of view (including the patient's) is seen as an opportunity to open dialogue and positively challenge and reflect on personal, societal and organisational values, attitudes and behaviours.

The drive to EBP is a highly desirable aspect of modern health services. However, it has been argued that it has minimised the role that values have in care delivery (Woodbridge and Fulford, 2004). It is rare that the evidence base for practice comes 'value free' (Fulford and Stanghellini, 2008). It is argued, therefore, that the drive for clinical quality through EBP must be delivered with a drive for values too (McGonagle et al., 2015).

Incorporating sources of evidence from patients, the public and carers into the delivery of care has a long tradition within nursing and underpins the ethos of holistic care. Their inclusion in research is also now recognised as essential (see www.invo.org.uk/ for guidance on how to involve the public in health and social care research). This aspect is explored further in Chapter 3. However, this source of evidence has its own inherent complexities and can be challenging. When research findings promoting the view that a specific form of intervention is most appropriate (for example, the use of a particular medication in managing mental health problems) are at odds with the service user's experience (the medication has specific side effects that make the person unwilling to take it), the clinical expertise of the nurse is essential in identifying the most appropriate course of action.

Institutional cultures, social and professional networks, evaluations such as 360-degree feedback and local/national policies are some of the forms of evidence found in the local setting (Rycroft-Malone et al., 2004a). Other relevant local evidence includes audits and individual patient preferences and service evaluations.

There are also some 'ready-made' forms of evidence available, where best evidence has been collected and summarised for use by healthcare professionals. Clinical Knowledge Summaries, produced by The National Institute for Health and Care Excellence (NICE) are an example of this type of resource. This is an online collection of concise summaries of available evidence, providing recommendations on how to manage commonly encountered clinical situations in care settings (see http://cks.nice.org.uk/#?char=A).

A further new initiative is the publication of BITEs (Brokering Innovation Through Evidence), which have been developed by the Collaboration for Leadership in Applied Health Research and Care (CLAHRC) as a means of conveying the 'need to know' information about a piece of research to busy clinicians and health and social care staff (see www.clahrcpp.co.uk/#!bites/c19df).

A relatively new initiative in EBP is that of **care bundles**. Here, elements of best practice evidence (usually between three and five) are grouped together in relation to a particular condition, treatment and/or procedure. These elements are ones that are generally used in practice but not necessarily applied in the same way or combination to all appropriate patients. Care bundles 'tie' together these elements into a unit that is delivered to every patient in the same way. Dawson and Endacott (2011) identified that combining elements in this way has a more positive impact on treatment outcomes than any one single element. They suggested that care bundles appear to be more effective than clinical guidelines in improving possible outcomes, as the former are seen as mandatory while the latter are often viewed as purely advisory.

Care bundles were originally developed in 2002 at the Johns Hopkins University in the USA in relation to critical care environments. It was found that using four interventions with patients on ventilators significantly reduced length of stay and number of ventilator days. Care bundles have now also been developed in a number of other areas, such as infection control, and are advocated by the Department of Health as a tool for high impact change. However, the then Institute for Healthcare Improvement (2012) warned against an ad hoc approach to bringing elements of care together, stressing that the strength of the bundles lies in the underpinning science, the way it is delivered and consistency in its application.

QUESTIONS

Having identified what counts as good evidence, the next task is to find the evidence. This requires the formulating of a relevant question, often considered the backbone of EBP. Ideas in relation to questions about practice can come from a range of situations, reflection on practice issues, audit outcomes and discussions between nurses, patients and/or other health professionals. Often, such questions are broad and unfocused, but if appropriate answers are to be found, then there is a need to develop specific, focused research questions.

Activity 2.3

You are currently working in a residential care setting. Mary, a 66-year-old patient in your care, has fallen and fractured her femur. In discussion with the rest of the care staff it is identified that there have been a number of falls over the year that have resulted in fractured femurs. Someone remembers reading about 'hip protectors' as a method of reducing injuries. You have been asked to look for some evidence to help make decisions as to how to address the issues. Where would you start?

An obvious starting place might be to go online and Google the words 'fractured femur', but this is likely to produce thousands of hits or nothing at all. There is a need to focus the search to ensure that the relevant information is obtained while vital pieces of information are not missed.

Activity 2.3

Stillwell et al. (2010) identified two forms of questions that practitioners might ask – **background** and **foreground**. **Background questions** are generally broad and have two parts:

1. The question's stem – who, what, where, when, how, why?
2. The area of clinical interest.

A background question might look something like 'What is the best way of treating depression?' There is a need to ask background questions, particularly for students and those new to an area of practice, in order to gain the knowledge and expertise needed in relation to a specific area. The problem with background questions is their broadness, which makes it difficult to find specific information, and searching for information is often done in a haphazard way – indeed, it is easy to end up looking in the wrong place.

Foreground questions ask about specific issues and are looking for particular knowledge. A foreground question might be something like 'Which is more effect in treating depression – cognitive behavioural therapy or medication?'

It is essential that a foreground question is formulated containing all the key elements for consideration, before searching the literature in relation to a particular issue. The question will be central to ensuring that the search is not too broad, which in turn may result in retrieving an overwhelming amount of literature, or too narrow in scope, resulting in key items being missed. There are a number of formats that can be used to help to create a search question; a commonly used one being **PICO** (see Table 2.4).

Table 2.4   Outline of PICO

Population	Intervention	Comparison	Outcome
Include 1. Disease/condition (e.g. cancer, schizophrenia) 2. Population (e.g. age) and setting (e.g. community)	Type of activity/ procedure/treatment or action, e.g. • use of a specific assessment tool • particular type of wound dressing • using a particular approach such as cognitive behavioural therapy	Alternative activities or actions against which comparisons are made between interventions. Sometimes this might be usual treatment.	Results of a specified action. All possible outcomes are explored.

As shown in Table 2.4:

P = population and could be something like adult males with depression.

I = intervention and could be something like cognitive behavioural therapy (CBT).

C = comparison and could be something like antidepressant medication.

O = outcome and could be something like raised mood.

The PICO question would then be:

In adult male service users diagnosed with depression is CBT more effective than antidepressants in raising mood?

In some instances the use of an extra letter such as T is added, which relates to the time frame over which the intervention would be observed, making PICOT. In the above question, for example, 'over a period of 18 months' could be added. In other instances the letter S is added, giving the acronym PICOS, with the S = Study type, providing the opportunity to limit the type of study to be included in the search of literature. In this case only RCTs might be considered.

Activity 2.4

Consider the above scenario about Mary, and apply the PICO principles. What question do you think would enable you to search for appropriate evidence? It might look something like this:

In female adults over the age of 65 years, is the use of hip protection more effective than normal precautions in reducing the incidence of fractured femurs following a fall?

The PICO framework tends to be most useful when asking 'effectiveness' questions and reflects the quantitative approach to research. However, it is less helpful for considering qualitative aspects of care such as patient experiences. The JBI offers an alternative formation – PICo:

Participants

phenomena of Interest

Context

If in relation to the above scenario the actual interest was in patients' experience of wearing hip protectors, the question in this instance might be:

In female adults over the age of 65 years (P), what is their experience of wearing hip protectors (I) in a hospital setting (Co)?

Formulating questions in this way allows focus on the real question that needs to be addressed and helps to move to the next stage of the process, searching for the evidence. The question will provide the key terms to be used in the search.

Activity 2.5

Think about a recent clinical experience and identify a patient whose care you were closely involved with. Focusing on one clinical intervention you undertook in relation to this person (giving an injection, attending to hygiene needs, involvement of patients in recreational/therapeutic activities), write a reflective account identifying:

(Continued)

(Continued)

1. What knowledge you were using during the intervention/activity, considering what areas of knowledge you felt most comfortable with and those that you need to develop further.
2. What evidence you used to direct how you organised your intervention/activity.
3. The questions you would ask if you wanted to find further evidence to support your practice in this area.

RESEARCH GOVERNANCE AND ETHICS

Anyone undertaking research needs to be aware of the principles of research ethics and governance. This is discussed in more detail in Chapter 6. Essentially, in the UK, The Health Research Authority (HRA) and the Devolved UK Administrations have developed a UK Policy Framework for Health and Social Care Research which sets out the high-level principles of good practice in the management and conduct of health and social care research in the UK, as well as the responsibilities that underpin high-quality ethical research (HRA, 2018). A core standard for healthcare organisations is that they have systems to ensure the principles and requirements of this research governance framework are consistently applied. As such, in the UK, all NHS organisations will have a Research Governance Department, which is an essential port of call for any employees looking to undertake research. Research governance departments will offer advice on the process for applying for ethical approval both locally and, where needed, nationally through the NHS integrated research application system (see www.myresearchproject.org.uk/).

Researchers have a responsibility to explain and justify their activities – to convey to others that their area of enquiry is both important and necessary and how they decide upon the focus of their research (Moule et al., 2016). Systems of governance and ethical approval are essential to this process, particularly in providing scrutiny over any potential for harm to those who take part in research.

Summary

*   Knowledge is broadly categorised into two types – propositional (formal) and non-propositional (personal) – and comes from three sources – tenacity, authority and a priori. Clinical knowledge can be seen as based on superstition, folklore, craft or science.

- Science is a body of knowledge organised in a systematic way based on observation, experiment and measurement.
- Evidence is information or data that supports or refutes beliefs in relation to a particular area of interest.
- Evidence on which to base clinical practice is best drawn from a variety of credible sources reflecting the multifaceted and complex needs of delivering care. There are four types of evidence on which nurses and other healthcare professionals can base their practice – research, clinical experience, service user/carer perspectives and local context.
- There are 'ready-made' forms of evidence available, where best evidence has been collected and summarised, such as clinical guidelines and summaries.
- Appropriate, focused questions are the backbone of EBP. The PICO format is helpful in the development of questions related to effectiveness, PICo for those related to feasibility, meaning and appropriateness.
- All clinical staff involved in research must familiarise themselves with local and national principles of research governance and ethics application processes.

FURTHER READING

Carper, B. (1978) 'Fundamental patterns of knowing in nursing', *Advances in Nursing Science*, 1: 13–23. This article is recommended for a full exploration of the nature of nursing knowledge.
Dawson, D. and Endacott, R. (2011) 'Implementing quality initiatives using a bundled approach', *Intensive Critical Care Nursing*, 27: 117–20. This article gives an overview of the development of care bundles.
Health Research Authority (HRA) (2018) *UK Policy Framework for Health and Social Care Research*. Health Research Authority.
Stillwell, S.B., Fineout-Overholt, E., Melnyk, B.M. and Williamson, K.M. (2010) 'Asking the clinical question: a key step in evidence-based practice', *American Journal of Nursing*, 110(3): 58–61. This article further explores the use of PICO in question formation.

USEFUL WEBLINKS

Clinical Knowledge Summaries: provides concise summaries of evidence related to common primary care issues and gives recommendations for practice. http://cks.nice.org.uk/#?char=A

The Health Research Authority (HRA): a body of the Department of Health in the UK, set up to protect and promote the interests of patients and the public in health and social care research. It has published or made available a number of key resources about good research practice. www.hra.nhs.uk/planning-and-improving-research/policies-standards-legislation/uk-policy-framework-health-social-care-research

NHS Evidence: enables users to simultaneously search 150 data sources for resources such as clinical summaries, guidelines, research literature, the British National Formulary. www.evidence.nhs.uk

Trip Database: a search engine that identifies high-quality evidence for use in clinical practice. www.tripdatabase.com

3

Service User and Carer Involvement

Paul Linsley and Janet Barker

Learning Outcomes

By the end of the chapter, you will be able to:

- discuss the issues related to patient involvement;
- consider appropriate ways of incorporating the patient's perspective into decision-making processes;
- develop and use appropriate resources to facilitate shared decision-making processes

INTRODUCTION

Modern healthcare has been defined in terms of four precepts: that it should be evidence based; patient–centred and inclusive of carers and the community; continuous and coordinated across settings; and ethically sound and regulated (Petrova et al., 2006). With this in mind, the following chapter highlights the importance of service user and carer involvement in the implementation of EBP. For service users, EBP lacks relevance and trustworthiness unless it explicitly factors in the expertise of service users themselves (Davies and Gray, 2016). UK policy recommends that service users and carers should be involved in all publicly funded health and social care research and that their contribution be recognised accordingly. Any attempt to judge the quality of health services would be incomplete without considering the experiences of people who access and use them (NICE, 2011). The terms 'service user' and 'carer' cover a broad range of people, and refer to those, who in one way or another, use, or are affected by, health and social care services. Increasingly, we are seeing the expression 'expert by experience' being used to define service user and carer involvement. Experts by experience are people who have personal experience of using or caring for someone who uses health or social care services (Care Quality Commission, 2018). The term can be defined as involving:

> The active participation of people who, because they have used services, can bring their knowledge and experience to contribute to the design, planning, delivery and evaluation of services at a local, regional and national level. (Scottish Executive 2006: 2)

The term 'experts by experience' emphasises the value that individuals with experiential knowledge bring to not only their own care and treatment but also that of others in a similar position. Within practice and research, we are increasingly seeing the use of 'experts' being put at the forefront of thinking.

Activity 3.1

Before reading any more of this chapter be sure to visit the Health Foundation website on patient-centred care at the following web address: www.health. org.uk/publication/person-centred-care-made-simple. Make sure to explore the site and record your observations and comments. Reflect on your practice as part of this.

The NMC (2018a) clearly outlines in its Code of Conduct the expectation that nurses will work collaboratively with patients, and Coulter and Collins (2011) have stated that health professionals are ethically obligated to discuss treatment options with patients and determine their individual preferences. In practice, this type of involvement is typified in **shared decision making** (SDM) whereby clinicians, patients and their carers make an informed decision together using the best available evidence and based upon both clinical need and patient preferences (Elwyn et al., 2010). SDM and support for self-management refer to a set of attitudes, roles and skills, supported by tools and organisational systems, which put patients and carers into a full partnership relationship with clinicians in all clinical interactions (Royal College of Physicians, 2013).

There is a potential tension between EBP as a scientific approach to care – based on sound evidence – and the underlying health philosophy of care being patient–centred, requiring nursing in particular to respond holistically to the individual needs of patients. However, Sidani et al. (2006) suggested the two approaches are complementary as both aim at ensuring that care is acceptable to the patient and delivered in the most effective way. Research suggests that active and embedded participation based on partnership working is most effective at achieving lasting change and can have positive effects on decision-making processes and staff attitudes and behaviour (see Box 3.1).

Box 3.1 The benefits to shared decision making have been identified as:

- People both receiving and delivering care can understand what is important to the other person.
- People feel supported and empowered to make informed choices and reach a shared decision about care.
- Health and social care professionals can tailor the care or treatment to the needs of the individual.

Source: NICE (2018).

Activity 3.2

Reflect on a recent experience in practice where changes have been made to a patient's care regime. How much involvement did the patient have in the decision processes? Could this be improved and if so how? Could you identify the evidence base on which the intervention was made?

Patients and their carers expect to be involved in decisions related to their health treatment options and care, and 'bring different but equally important forms of expertise to the decision-making process' (Coulter and Collins, 2011: 2). The professionals' expertise lies in their knowledge of the disease processes and treatment options available; the patients bring their experience and understanding of the impact of the disease on their everyday lives and their personal preference, attitudes and values.

There are certain characteristics associated with SDM, these are:

- the sharing of information between at least two individuals;
- all parties making and agreeing the decision;
- an ongoing partnership between the patient and the clinical team.

Best and Hagen (2010) proposed that the approach involves working collaboratively with patients by:

- listening to and exploring what a patient knows about their health problems and care needs;
- providing opportunities to express concerns and worries;
- discussing possible treatment options;

- providing appropriate information about these options;
- making sure information is understood;
- ensuring decisions reflect patient's wishes;
- offering regular opportunities to review decisions.

Involving patients in decision making assumes that they are motivated and have the power and ability to be involved in decisions made about their healthcare. In reality, some patients want to be more involved than others. It is suggested that younger people and those people with higher educational levels often want to take a more active role in decisions made about their care. However, it is possible that a preference for an active role in healthcare decisions may be a personality trait rather than a group-specific characteristic. Therefore, it is important to check all patients' preferred level of involvement.

> **Activity 3.3**
>
> Consider your current areas of practice and identify patients who appear to want to be involved in the decision process and those who do not. What might be the reasons for these differences?

In a landmark study of its kind, the Department of Health document *Building on the Best: Choice, Responsiveness and Equity in the NHS* (2003) reported on a consultation of over 110,000 people and identified that people want to be involved in the decisions made about their health and healthcare. The type of experience patients want from the NHS was defined as:

- getting good treatment in a comfortable, caring and safe environment, delivered in a calm and reassuring way;
- having information to make choices, to feel confident and to feel in control;
- being talked to and listened to as an equal; being treated with honesty, respect and dignity.

Patient preferences and experiences can be garnered in two ways – from individual patients or collations of multiple sources. There are a number of possible ways in which to gather a general understanding of collated patient preferences. These can give a general insight into how patients view certain aspects of care; what might influence uptake of treatment and the continuation of treatment regimens; and the factors that lead to dissatisfaction. This information can also be useful when discussing options with individual patients as it can provide a background for discussions and exploring specific issues that may be of concern to individuals. It can also provide a source of information to include in your decision-making processes, by identifying possible issues you may need to take into consideration that individual patients have not identified.

There now exist a number of ways to think about service user involvement. One of the best-known approaches to thinking about patients and carers is the 'Ladder of Participation', developed by Sherry Arnstein (1969).

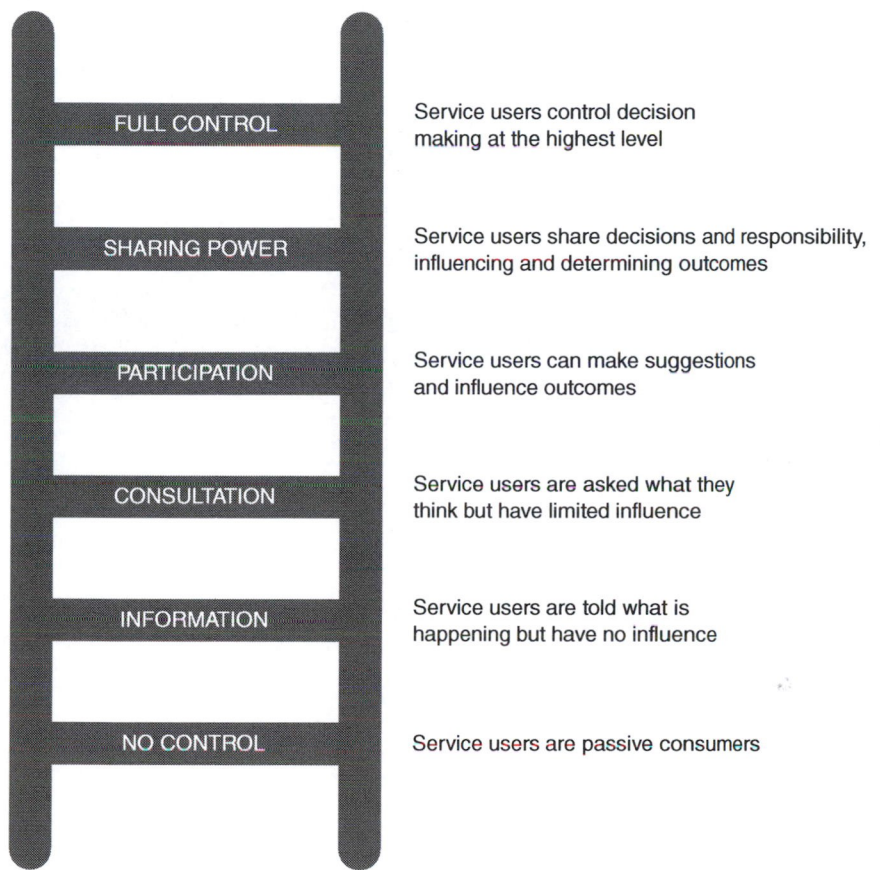

FULL CONTROL — Service users control decision making at the highest level

SHARING POWER — Service users share decisions and responsibility, influencing and determining outcomes

PARTICIPATION — Service users can make suggestions and influence outcomes

CONSULTATION — Service users are asked what they think but have limited influence

INFORMATION — Service users are told what is happening but have no influence

NO CONTROL — Service users are passive consumers

Figure 3.1   Ladder of Participation

Source: Adapted by the Offender Health Collaborative (2015).

Interventions that promote involvement can then be targeted at the different levels. This Ladder of Participation can be thought of in terms of individual, group or community involvement. The model enables clinicians, as well as researchers and administrators, to think about how they might go about promoting service user involvement at the different levels, as well as evaluate their effects on working practices and organisational responses to the needs of service users and their carers.

Patients and their families will have expectations about how they will be treated and of the type of service they will receive. Patient expectation is what the patient expects according to available resources. This will be based on their understanding of their illness or condition and will have been formed over time. Conventional news sources, internet sites and community and individual values and beliefs also influence patient expectation. A patient's understanding depends not only on the material that they receive but also on how the patient assimilates that information and translates it into actionable beliefs. Patients struggle to comprehend a service when there is a gap between what the patient expects and how they perceive the service. To a large extent, people will judge a service as either being good or bad based on whether it has met their expectations regardless of them getting better or being provided with the support they need.

INVOLVING PATIENTS IN SDM

Gaining a patient's perspective requires giving full attention to the individual's 'narrative' – their story – and enabling them to freely express their beliefs, values and concerns in a non-judgemental and supportive way. This requires good communication and interpersonal skills and the ability to build a trusting relationship with the patient. The process of SDM, as identified by Simon et al. (2006), includes several steps:

- Recognition that a decision needs to be made;
- Identification of partners in the process as equals;
- Statement of the options as equal;
- Exploration of understanding and expectations;
- Identifying preferences;
- Negotiating options/concordance;
- Sharing the decision; and
- Arranging follow-up to evaluate decision-making outcomes.

Kitson (2002) suggests there are basic skills underpinning this activity:

- Knowing what questions to ask;
- Using active listening skills;
- Having an awareness of the principles underpinning patient-centred care;
- Putting the principles of patient-centred care into practice;
- Being open to new ideas and alternative ways of thinking;
- Making explicit links between different sources of knowledge, evidence and decision-making processes.

These basic skills were expanded upon by Siminoff (2012), who proposed the following steps when engaging with patients and their families in SDM.

- Access patient and family understanding of their symptoms and illness and listen to their explanations.

- Validate patient and family concerns.
- Iteratively check understanding by asking patients to explain or 'teach back' to you, in their own words, what you have just explained.
- Use relational communication strategies to build rapport and shared meaning. While words are used to convey information, how they are used along with their corresponding non-verbal cues also communicates significant meaning. Consider not only what patients are saying but also what they may not be saying and always confirm to avoid misunderstanding and conflict. Be cognisant of non-verbal cues and the messages being sent as a result.
- Discuss sources of information. Encourage patients to talk about what they have learned or know about their illness and about their source(s) for that information. Encouraging patients to share can allow you to reinforce pertinent information while dispelling any inaccurate or incorrect information. It is critically important that misinformation is addressed in a non-judgemental way so that the conversation continues, and patients do not feel belittled. Acknowledge and legitimate that patients may continue to function under a different explanatory paradigm. Understanding and accepting this difference allows you to work as effectively as possible with the patient.
- Consider how to incorporate patient values and needs in treatment plans. Ask patients what they hope to accomplish with treatment and what preferences or suggestions for treatment they may have. Engage the patient in a discussion of the pros and cons of treatment(s) and have them relate them to their values and needs as appropriate and participate in shared decision making.

Assessing individual preferences from patients in your care and attempting to integrate patient preferences into clinical decisions is central to EBP. Sidani et al. (2006) identify this as a three-step process:

1. Identifying evidence on which to base care, accounting for alternative approaches to meet patient needs and preparing easy to understand descriptions of the evidence.
2. Informing patients of the possible options and identifying preferences.
3. Integrating patient preferences into the delivery of care.

As step 1 indicates, it is essential that you have the full information regarding the proposed intervention(s) so you can ensure the patient has a complete understanding of the issues. Careful thought and attention needs to be given to the type of information provided to patients. The DISCERN initiative provides a tool to access the quality and type of information given to patients to aid decision making in clinical practice.

Visit the DISCERN website at www.discern.org.uk. Compare the information you provide to patients with the type recommended by DISCERN.

Activity 3.4

CONSENT AND CAPACITY

Legislation relating to consent, mental capacity and competency is central to patient involvement and decision making, and therefore must be considered when involving patients in SDM. The NMC (2018a) emphasises that patients have the right to be involved in all aspects of decision making and that nurses have a duty to obtain consent before any care is given. It also stipulates that individuals have the right to accept or refuse treatment and their decisions should be respected and supported. However, the Mental Capacity Act (MCA) (DH, 2005) may have implications for certain aspects of consent in specific circumstances, particularly where health issues may impact on capacity to consent to treatment or an individual has learning disabilities.

The MCA (DH, 2005) allows for others to make decisions if the patient's capacity to do so is compromised through mental ill-health, learning disabilities (intellectual disabilities), drink, drugs, pain, fear, or the effects of physical diseases. A person's capacity to consent may fluctuate, temporarily or permanently, or may relate to certain aspects of care – individuals may have the capacity to make certain decisions, but not others. However, it must not be automatically assumed that people do not have the capacity to make decisions; the default position is always that 'a person is assumed to have capacity unless it is established that he lacks capacity' (DH, 2005: section 1(2)).

The MCA also stipulates that someone must not be considered incapable until all possible ways of helping the person have been explored. It stresses that capacity should not be confused with the health professional's view of the reasonableness of a decision (i.e. that a particular choice is seen as unwise from a professional perspective). Where capacity is in doubt a full assessment must be carried out which considers the individual's ability to:

- understand information relevant to the decision;
- retain the information;
- weigh up information as part of the decision-making process;
- communicate effectively – verbally, sign language or muscle movement such as blinking.

The MCA clearly outlines the processes that must be in place before someone is considered not to have the capacity to be involved in decisions about their healthcare.

STANDARDISED PATIENT DECISION AIDS

Standardised **patient decision aids** (PDAs) are available to help facilitate patient decision making. These tools are usually generated following clinical research and studies of patients' information needs and guide patients through the decision-making process (O'Connor et al., 2004). PDAs have been well researched in some areas (such as breast cancer treatment) and less so in others (such as in mental health). Nevertheless, there is a growing body of research round these approaches. It is intended that they will be used when there is more than one possible option available in relation to a particular health issue. Each PDA presents the various risks and benefits of each option in a clear and simple way, enabling the patient to make an informed choice based on their own preferences and values. Many include ways of clarifying individuals' values and take patients through the decision process step-by-step.

PDAs come in many forms – leaflets, interactive software, workbooks – and are intended to be used by health professionals and patients to inform their discussions rather than replace them. They do, however, provide information in a format that patients can consider at their own pace and in their own time, and then return to in the discussions of options with health professionals. It is suggested that the PDAs do three things:

1. Provide an overview of the facts relating to the intervention option.
2. Help people to clarify their preferences and values.
3. Provide a means of communicating these to health professionals.

The Cochrane Review Team of Patient Decision Aids creates and reviews decision aids; a register of these can be found on the Collaboration's site: www.cochrane.org/CD001431/COMMUN_decision-aids-help-people-who-are-facing-health-treatment-or-screening-decisions

Involving patients in decision making is not without its problems. As Lanfear et al. (2011) identified, a person's level of self-confidence may affect their willingness to participate in decision making. There is a potential for power struggles if the patient's preference runs counter to what professionals think is the most effective or feasible treatment or chooses an option that is thought to be detrimental to their wellbeing. Michaels et al. (2008) cautioned that tensions can arise if patients reject professionals' recommendations. Equally, there may be difficulties in relation to a patient's perspectives and that of their family members, who, believing they have their loved ones' best interests at heart, advocate different approaches to treatment.

SDM IN THE MENTAL HEALTH SETTING

The advent of the 'recovery' model in mental health, which emphasises the importance of incorporating service users' values and preferences in the delivery of care, would seem to indicate that the adoption of SDM is essential. The recovery model advocates the need to empower service users and promotes collaboration between professionals, the carers and the individual. SDM in mental health has been shown to improve adherence to treatment regimens and service user satisfaction (Drake et al., 2012) and research in this area is growing. However, as Adams et al. (2007) identified, service users frequently feel they are not involved in decision-making processes and Deegan and Drake (2006) noted there is a need for more work in this area, calling for the development of PDAs specifically designed to support people with mental health problems.

There are specific barriers to SDM in mental health:

- The traditional use of a medical/disease focused treatment model.
- Mental health professionals' legal and moral obligation to the service user and society to prevent harm to self and/or others.

- Expectations of others – professional agencies and informal carers.
- Service users' competence, insight and mental state.

Despite these issues, increasingly, service users, their carers and mental health professionals are looking for ways to promote SDM.

The National Institute for Health and Care Excellence (2009) has advocated the use of **'advanced decisions'** in mental health settings, for people with schizophrenia to overcome issues related to competency to make decisions due to mental health problems. Such advanced decisions are legally binding under the MCA (DH, 2005) if they are seen as valid (the individual had capacity to make the decision at the time and has not expressed a change in opinion) and applicable (the need for treatment has come into effect and the individual is incapable of making the decision at that time).

Sidley (2012) suggested that for people with complex and/or severe mental health problems advanced decisions can help to shape future treatment and is likely to have a positive impact on therapeutic outcomes. Service users and care providers often have different perspectives as to what are priorities in care and what represents a good outcome. For example, Deegan and Drake (2006) discussed the perspectives people with mental health problems may have in relation to medications – such as the side effects being worse than the illness experience or there is only a need to take medication when they are experiencing distress. Practitioners are said to be more concerned with the effectiveness of medications in reducing symptoms of mental illness and preventing relapses. They advocate that anything that facilitates communication and offers involvement is likely to have a positive effect on patient recovery and see advanced directives as part of the shared decision-making process.

Involving mental health service users and their families in their care can make a huge difference in the lives of people – improving the quality and impact of services on offer, contributing to wider outcomes and enabling service users to build a new identity that supports their recovery journey. Increasingly, there is a focus on co-production of knowledge and services between parties. Co-production has been defined as:

> A way of working whereby citizens and decision makers, or people who use services, family carers and service providers work together to create a decision or service which works for them all. The approach is value driven and built on the principle that those who use a service are best placed to help design it. (National Occupational Standards, 2013)

Furthermore,

> Co-production is not just a word, it is not just a concept, it is a meeting of minds coming together to find a shared solution. In practice, it involves people who use services being consulted, included and working together from the start to the end of any project that affects them. (Service user quote from the Think Local Act Personal (2011) campaign)

Co-production has been broken down into the following (Löffler, 2009):

- Co-design, including planning of services;

- Co-decision making in the allocation of resources;
- Co-delivery of services, including the role of volunteers in providing the service;
- Co-evaluation of the service.

It is important to stress the difference between co-production and participation: participation means being consulted while co-production means being equal partners and co-creators. All involvement should be meaningful and pursued with purpose.

SDM IN CHILD HEALTH

Including children in the decision-making process is particularly complex and often requires consideration of the child's developmental stage and parental responsibility. Griffith and Tengnah (2012) identified three developmental stages:

1. Tender years – where the child is considered not to have decision-making competency, therefore decisions are made by whoever has parental responsibility for the child.
2. Gillick competent – where a child under the age of 16 years is assessed in terms of their maturity (experiences and ability to manage influences such as peer pressure) and intelligence (understanding and ability to weigh up the various benefits and risks and long-term impact of decisions). The more serious the decision, the greater the level of competency required.
3. Young persons – where 16- and 17-year-old individuals are allowed to consent and participate in decisions as if they were at the age of consent.

It is expected that children will be involved in the decision-making process at the level appropriate for their age, ability and experience (Coyne et al., 2011). Children with long-term illnesses are felt to have a high level of competence in making decisions. It is suggested that children feel more valued and less anxious when involved in decision processes, and it is expected that health professionals are at least aware of and include children's views in making decisions about their care (Baston, 2008). Providing children with age-appropriate information – for example, using play or dolls – enables them to cope better with their illness. However, as decision making involves three parties (child, parents and health professional) it can be particularly problematic.

Where parents are involved in decision making it has been found that the level of desired involvement can range from 'none' where this is seen as the nurse/doctor's role, to providing comfort, to acting as the child's advocate and having primary responsibility for making decisions (Franck et al., 2012). These seem to reflect the positions adopted by patients in terms of their preferred level of involvement in decision making.

Moore and Kirk (2010) identified a number of the factors that can enhance children's participation in decision making; an overview of these is provided in Box 3.2.

Box 3.2   Enhancement of child involvement in decision making

- Presence of parent.
- Parents' approval of child's participation.
- Parents with a good standard of education.
- Child has a good understanding and knowledge about their condition.
- Child has the ability to access information about their illness.
- Age and maturity of child.
- Experienced healthcare professionals.

Activity 3.5

Consider your own area of practice and identify what is available to facilitate children's involvement in decision making about their care. How could this be improved?

SDM IN THE LEARNING DISABILITIES SETTING

Valuing People: A New Strategy for the 21st Century (DH, 2001) was the first White Paper for 30 years which specifically addressed the care of people with learning disabilities (LD). It had four central principles, which would seem to reflect the SDM ethos:

1. Choice.
2. Independence.
3. Rights.
4. Inclusion.

However, various reports (such as *Healthcare for All: Report of the Independent Inquiry into Access to Healthcare for People with Learning Disabilities* [DH, 2008]) have demonstrated that people with learning disabilities continue to experience inequalities in the quality of care they receive. Most damning was the report *Death by Indifference* (Mencap, 2007), which described the deaths of six people with LD while receiving care in the NHS, and attributed this to institutional discrimination against people with LD and a belief that they are not capable of being involved in decisions about their care. More recent reports (*The Learning Disabilities Mortality Review* (LeDeR) Programme (2017) and the *Confidential Inquiry into Premature Deaths of People with Learning Disabilities (CIPOLD)* [Heslop et al., 2013]) have echoed these findings.

No Voice Unheard, No Right Ignored – A Consultation for People with Learning Disabilities, Autism and Mental Health Conditions (DH, 2015) and *Valuing People Now* (DH, 2007b) identified the need for people with LD to be in charge and to have greater choice and control over their lives and support to develop person-centred plans. However, it has also been shown that many healthcare professionals lack confidence in working with this group of people and limited understanding of their needs (Barr and Sowney, 2007). Both CIPOLD (Heslop et al., 2013) and LeDeR (2017) have identified the need for further education for healthcare staff.

There are a number of ways through which people with learning disabilities can be involved in decision making, such as:

- gathering information from family/carers and friends with regard to the ways that the person communicates/responds to specific situations and undertakes daily activities;
- developing individual support packages. This may mean providing information in picture form, using videos or using symbols;
- identifying ways to facilitate meaningful communication such as 'Intensive Interaction' (Nind and Hewett, 2006). See www.intensiveinteraction.org for further information;
- providing accessible information. See www.england.nhs.uk/ourwork/accessibleinfo/ for further information.

As with mental health, Learning Disability services have embraced the idea of co-production. If we really are to meet the needs of people that we support, then our intent to involve them should be made on a genuine basis.

INVOLVING THE SERVICE USER AND THEIR CARER IN RESEARCH

Involving people with lived experience in health research brings with it a number of benefits, including improved recruitment and retention in studies and better communication of findings to target groups (Domecq et al., 2014). The experiential knowledge of living with a condition ensures that findings are contextualised and timely and can add relevance and credibility to the research (Thompson et al., 2009). It is argued here that not to include service users and their carers in research could be said to be unethical, not least because those with experience of mental and physical health difficulties should have a say in research that is about them and has an impact on them, but also because involving those from the target population in the research design may help ensure that the study is conducted ethically and sensitively.

There are a number of ways in which people can become involved in the research process. The National Institute for Health Research (NIHR) (2010: 2) identified five principal stages of research where user involvement should be considered in all studies. These stages are:

- the development of the grant application;
- the design and management of the research;
- the undertaking of the research;
- the analysis of the research data;
- the dissemination of research findings.

The NIHR (2010: 2) also identified three levels of service–user involvement, these being:

- consultation – whereby the researcher asks users for their views and advice on certain aspects of the research;
- collaboration – whereby the researcher and service user work together to make decisions about the research;
- user led or controlled – whereby the service user makes the decisions about the research, for example what is to be researched and how the study is conducted.

While service user-led research can be seen as a significant development within the research community, much of service user involvement remains at the consultation level of engagement. The challenge, particularly with service user-led or controlled research is how best to retain its honesty and avoid the twin dangers of either becoming a tokenistic exercise or being seen as a panacea (McLaughlin, 2010).

Activity 3.6

Ferguson and Day (2007) identified that novice nurses have difficulty in identifying patient preferences and values. Complete a SWOT analysis (refer to Appendix 1) and identify your future learning needs in this area.

Summary

- Involving experts by experience in the decisions is central to EBP, affecting adherence to treatment and patient satisfaction.
- Patient preferences and experiences can be gleaned in two ways – from individual patients or collations of multiple sources.
- Patients may have different preferred levels of involvement. There is a need to check what level of involvement a patient wants in the decision-making process.
- The majority of patients, irrespective of the health issue, prefer a collaborative approach to decision making.
- There is a need to provide information for patients in a way that facilitates understanding of the issues under consideration.
- Standardised patient decision aids (PDAs) are available to help facilitate patient decision making.
- The Mental Capacity Act (DH, 2005) allows for others to make decisions, only if the patient's capacity to do so is compromised.

FURTHER READING

Davies, K. and Gray, M. (2016) 'The place of service-user expertise in evidence-based practice', *Journal of Social Work*, 17(1): 3–20.

National Institute for Health Research (NIHR) (2010) *Involving Users in the Research Process. A 'How to' Guide for Researchers*. London: NIHR.

NICE (2018) *Shared Decision Making*. www.nice.org.uk/about/what-we-do/our-programmes/nice-guidance/nice-guidelines/shared-decision-making. (accessed 23 July 2018).

Petrova, M., Dale, J. and Fulford, K.W.M. (2006) 'Values-based practice in primary care: easing the tensions between individual values, ethical principles and best evidence', *Br J Gen Pract*, 56 (530): 703–9.

USEFUL WEBLINKS

INVOLVE was established in 1996 and is part of, and funded by, the National Institute for Health Research, to support active public involvement in NHS, public health and social care research. www.invo.org.uk

4

Clinical Judgement and Decision Making

Paul Linsley and Janet Barker

Learning Outcomes

By the end of the chapter you will be able to:

- discuss the nature of clinical judgement and decision making;
- recognise the processes involved in clinical judgement and decision making;
- identify and use appropriate decision-making frameworks.

INTRODUCTION

Today, we live in a world of rapidly accelerating change brought about by the application of science and technology to almost every aspect of our daily lives. For a variety of reasons, the health professions have not always been able to keep up with these advances and integrate them readily into clinical practice. Health and social care communities continually produce large amounts of research leading to revised methods of treatment and care for patients; however, this research does not always translate into clinical practice nor changes to service delivery (Kristensen et al., 2016). Associated with this problem of providing for change is the increasing concern that is being felt for effectiveness and efficiency in care and treatment planning and decision making. In order to bridge what has been termed this 'theory–practice gap' (Monaghan, 2015), any changes in thinking brought about by new research must eventually be made actionable and usable, and adapted to local practice, in order to produce the desired outcome over time. This often requires nurses and other healthcare professionals to take a lead in putting the evidence into practice and making the required changes. These demands entail an increasing degree of professionalism, as well as a framework within which decisions can be reached. EBP provides such a framework for decision making and this is one of the reasons why it is heavily promoted in the literature and by professional bodies the world over.

Portney (2004) suggested that EBP should more correctly be called evidence-based decision making, as it requires practitioners to draw on a range of information and decide as to what is actually required. Evidence-Based Decision Making has been described as 'a process for making decisions about a programme, practice, or policy that is grounded in the best available evidence and informed by experiential evidence from the field and relevant contextual evidence' (Jennings and Hall, 2011: 245). The idea is that 'good-quality decisions should be based on a combination of critical thinking and the best available evidence' (Barends et al., 2014). This approach stands in contrast to opinion-based decisions and the untested views and ideas of individuals or groups, 'often inspired by ideological standpoints, prejudices, or speculative conjecture' (Davies, 2004: 3). It has been suggested that evidence-based practice is mediated and actioned by an interplay between individuals, new knowledge and the actual context in which the evidence is to be operationalised and utilised as part of daily practice (Boaz et al., 2011). Furthermore, decisions concerned with care and treatment planning call for a deep understanding and concern for people and necessitate balancing the social and task requirements of the profession and organisation to which the nurse belongs.

Prior to the advent of EBP most health professionals based clinical decision making on 'their vast educational knowledge coupled with intelligent guesswork, hunches and experience' (Pape, 2003: 155). Reliance on such approaches is no longer seen as appropriate due to a number of factors, particularly over-confidence (Thompson et al., 2013). Clinical judgement and decision making are identified as central to clinical competence. Nursing not only involves knowing the how and why of delivering a certain type of care but also the ability to give sound rationales and justifications for clinical judgements and decisions taken. Melnyk and Fineout-Overholt (2018) have stated that it is useful to think of EBP as requiring clinicians to be involved in two essential activities regarding decision making – critically appraising evidence (discussed in Chapter 6) and using clinical judgement to consider how applicable the evidence is to their own area of practice.

In its simplest terms, decision making involves determining precise and concrete goals or objectives, and then selecting, from alternatives, a course of action that is most likely to lead to a successful outcome. However, decision making is not a straightforward activity. Clinical decisions are often characterised by situations of uncertainty where not all the information needed to make them is, or can be, known. It is also recognised that nurses and other healthcare professionals have become data inputters and not users of data and that there is an over-reliance on protocol rather than thinking through the situation at hand. The increasing complexity of the care needs of individuals, care interventions and care delivery settings require finely honed clinical judgement skills to ensure clinical decision making is of the highest standard. Lamb and Sevdalis (2011) have identified that clinical judgement and decision-making skills take practitioners beyond purely technical or knowledge-based skills, proposing these to be 'key non-technical' skills essential for the safe delivery of care.

Decisions of this kind also call for a great amount of creative and imaginative thinking and cover a wide range of activities.

Activity 4.1

Before reading any more of this chapter, answer the following questions: How do you put what you have read into practice? How does this affect the way in which you make clinical decisions?

WHAT IS CLINICAL JUDGEMENT?

As identified above, clinical judgement is an essential skill for all health professionals and one that separates them from undertaking a purely technical role. Various terms are used in relation to this activity (clinical reasoning, problem solving and critical thinking) but all are related to the ability to consider the various issues at hand, make a judgement in relation to the impact of the various elements and come up with a decision as to what is the appropriate action to take. A useful definition of clinical judgement is that proposed by Tanner (2006: 204) who defined it as the 'interpretation or conclusion about a patient's needs, concerns, or health problems, and/or the decision to take action (or not), use or modify standard approaches, or improvise new ones as deemed appropriate by the patient's responses'. Levett-Jones et al. (2010) suggested there are five 'rights' in relation to this concept – right cues, right patient, right action, right time for the right reason.

The important thing is to make structured decisions based on sound clinical judgement. Decisions will have implications for patient outcomes and as such must deserve serious consideration. The number and type of decisions that nurses and other healthcare professionals face are determined to some extent by their understanding and perception of their work, operational autonomy, and the degree to which they see themselves as active and influential decision makers. Thompson et al. (2001) identified that nurses made clinical decisions in six key areas:

1. Intervention/effectiveness: choosing between intervention X and intervention Y.
2. Targeting: these decisions relate to 'choosing which patient will benefit the most from this intervention'.
3. Timing: these commonly take the form of choosing the best time to deploy particular interventions.
4. Communication: these decisions focus on choices relating to ways of delivering and receiving information to and from patients, families and colleagues. Most often these decisions relate to the communication of risks and benefits of different interventions or prognostic categories.
5. Service organisation, delivery and management: decisions concerning the configuration or processes of service delivery.

6. Experimental, understanding or hermeneutic: these decisions relate to the interpretation of cues in the process of care. The choices involved might include deciding on the ways in which a patient may be experiencing a particular situation, and are intuitive to some extent.

Decision making is influenced not only by the available evidence but also by individual values, client choice, theories, ethics, legislation, regulation and healthcare resources (DiCenso et al., 2005). No decision, however, should ever be made without an accompanying judgement as to the appropriateness of that decision (van Graan and Williams, 2017).

> Reflect on a recent practice experience where a particular intervention appeared more appropriate for some patients than others. What factors impacted on the suitability of specific interventions for different individuals?
>
> **Activity 4.2**

> Can you identify any decisions that you made recently where you may not have been aware of why you made the decision? Reflect on why you made this decision and what influenced you.
>
> **Activity 4.3**

It is proposed that practitioners consider evidence in terms of its relevance and weight; however, this is an individual assessment, so what might be considered relevant and given greater weight by one clinician may not be considered in the same way by another (Lasater, 2011). In any two clinical situations the context and individual nurse's experience/ knowledge will impact on the judgements and decisions made. All clinical judgements have ethical considerations, with the health professional weighing up the potential benefits and risks involved in any decision made. Frequently there are a number of options available, each of which carries its own risks and benefits. This adds another dimension to the decision-making process, and often it is the patient's preferences that indicate which is the best choice of action (see Chapter 3). The relative stability and security provided by norms or tacit rules of interaction allow individuals in a given community to make more or less accurate predictions concerning the way others will behave and react in everyday life. However, to rely solely on this 'knowledge' for the purposes of decision making can lead to compliancy (and mistakes) and fails to recognise others as individuals.

The reasoning processes used in clinical judgement tend to be described as involving either analytical or intuitive activities (Tanner, 2006). The former involves the breaking down of a problem into its constituent parts, considering these, and weighing up the alternative approaches available in solving the problem. Usually, this involves the processing of scientific data. Intuitive processes are seen as drawing on inherent knowledge, skills and experiences to find the answer to the problem. These two options are often seen as the opposite poles of a continuum. However, the idea of a 'cognitive continuum' is possibly more helpful in understanding the processes involved as these two activities are not 'mutually exclusive' (Standing, 2017). Different approaches can be used in different situations depending on the complexity, ambiguity and presentation of the issue, and both may be necessary when dealing with uncertain situations. The more complex, familiar or urgent the issue the more likely you are to rely on intuition. Any combination of these three elements will result in the use of differing levels of analysis and/or intuition.

Activity 4.4

Identify and record:

- a situation where you have made a clinical decision on an emotional or biased basis;
- your actions as a result of this;
- the resulting care that followed.

Standing (2017) provided a cognitive continuum of clinical judgement in nursing based on identifying nine cognitive modes used by nurses in practice (see Table 4.1). No one mode is seen as more important than another; these simply reflected the types of knowledge drawn on in the clinical judgement and decision-making processes of nurses and the sort of activities nurses are likely to engage in. The intuitive mode is seen most frequently in face-to-face encounters with patients, whereas the experimental research mode is related to establishing effectiveness of intervention and is more distant from day-to-day care activities.

Table 4.1 Cognitive modes of nursing practice

Judgement process	Description
Intuitive	Drawing on tacit knowledge and arriving at a judgement without being aware of the process by which it was reached. Usually occurs in face-to-face care delivery situations.
Reflective	Incorporates both reflection in and on care delivery actions.
Patient and peer assisted	Encompasses seeking patient preferences and/or the expertise of other healthcare professionals.
System assisted	Involves the use of guidelines, problem-solving frameworks and decision aids.

Judgement process	Description
Critical review of evidence (experience and research)	Identification of relevant information and application of this to the current situation.
Action research and audit	Gathering information through implementing and evaluating changes to care delivery systems.
Qualitative research	Seeking to understand the patient's experience and inform future practice by undertaking qualitative research.
Survey research	Answering questions related to future care delivery by collecting data via surveys.
Experimental research	Testing the effectiveness of intervention through the use of experimental research designs such as RCTs.

It has been proposed that an over-reliance on intuition may give rise to problems associated with bias – an under- or over-estimation of the importance of certain factors or information. Bias in the form of stereotyping, prejudice or selective memory can influence how you perceive and respond to information and individual patients. Equally, basing judgements and decisions purely on personal experience and knowledge results in important research evidence being ignored or undervalued. Reliance on past experience while playing an important part in clinical decision making can also impede clinical judgement if not challenged in any way. Good decisions can only be evaluated against future events, while experience belongs to the past. This does not mean to say that experience is to be discounted, only that it is but one guide to action. Hammond (2007) identified that where analytical approaches to decision making are used errors occur infrequently but when they do they are often on a large scale; whereas errors resulting from intuition-based approaches occur frequently but tend to be small in nature. It is, therefore, essential that nurses and healthcare professionals can defend judgements and justify how they reached these and the decisions made.

WHAT IS CLINICAL DECISION MAKING?

Thompson and Stapley (2011) proposed that clinical judgement and clinical decision making are closely linked but separate concepts. The former is about an evaluation of a situation, and the latter is concerned with whether or not to take action and what type of action to take if necessary. For example, one might consider that a particular patient's diet is poor (judgement) and choose to provide them with an education package related to healthy eating (decision). Benner et al. (1996: 2) suggested that clinical judgement relates to 'the ways in which nurses come to understand the problems, issues, or concerns of clients/patients, to attend to salient information and to respond in concerned and involved ways'. In this way decision making is seen as an interaction between three things – the patient's preferences (discussed in Chapter 3); the evidence available on which to base practice; and the clinical judgement of the nurse involved based on personal experience and knowledge. These three components come together to produce a clinical decision as to what action should be taken – see Figure 4.1.

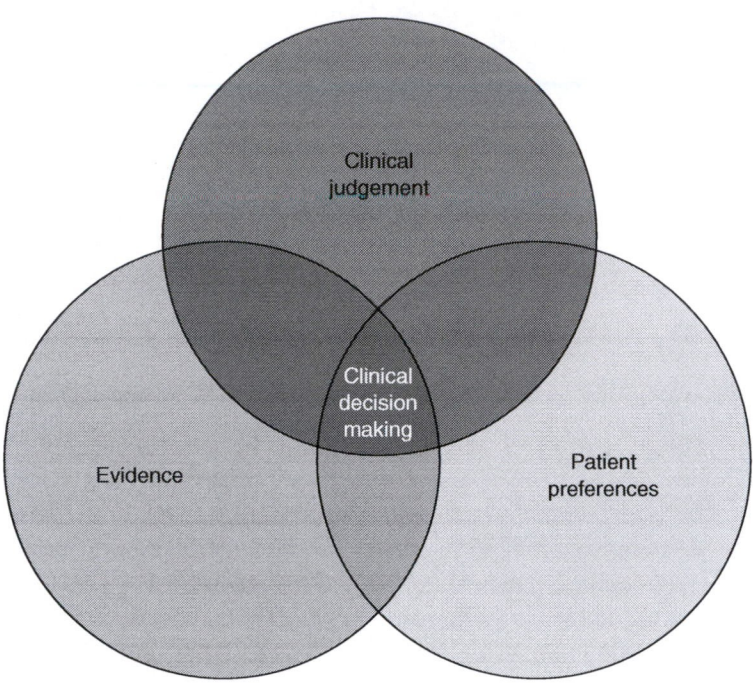

Figure 4.1   Components of clinical decision making

The core skills relating to good decision making have been identified as:

- Pattern recognition: learning from experience.
- Critical thinking: removing emotion from our reasoning, being 'sceptical', questioning and not taking things at face value, examining assumptions, being open-minded and receptive to change, and lastly being able to evaluate the evidence.
- Communication skills: active listening – listening to the patient, what they say, and what they don't say; and adopting and pursuing a patient-centred approach – the ability to provide information in a comprehensive way to allow patients, their carers and family to be involved in the decision–making process.
- Team work: using the gathered evidence to enlist help, support and advice from col– leagues and the wider multidisciplinary team.
- Sharing: learning and getting feedback from colleagues on your decision making.
- Reflection: using feedback from others and the outcomes of the decisions to reflect on the decisions that were taken in order to enhance practice delivery in the future. (Adapted from NHS Scottish Executive (2006))

Reflection is a central feature of clinical judgement and decision making as it requires health professionals to consider and make links between the evidence, their own knowledge, skills and experience and that of other team members as well as patient preferences, beliefs and values. However, for this to be effective in aiding clinical judgement it must be undertaken in a clear and structured way rather than simply 'thinking about' the issues. It has been identified that appropriate reflection and particularly reflective writing encourage the transfer of knowledge from one situation to another and help in knowledge transformation – consideration of the relevance current experiences may have for future activities (Nielsen et al., 2007). The reflective process is discussed in greater depth in Chapter 10.

> Consider the last clinical decision you made. How did you arrive at the decision? Were you aware of analysing the various aspects of the issue or was it reached more intuitively? Did you make the judgement and decision objectively, using all the data and evidence to hand? Did your personal attitudes or biases have a part to play in the decision? Did you involve the patient in the decision-making process – from the initial information gathering to agreeing a course of action? Examine your own decision-making patterns.

Activity 4.5

The nursing process of assess, plan, implement and evaluate requires quality decision making. For example, during the assessment phase of the cycle, increased knowledge on the part of the nurse leads to greater clinical currency and judgement. The more experienced nurse knows what to look for based upon clinical knowledge and personal experience and can use this information alongside the available evidence, policy and procedure to inform the care that they give. Evaluation ensures that decisions are reviewed and lessons are learnt. A good decision from an evidence-based perspective is one that successfully integrates four elements:

1. Professional expertise ('know–how' knowledge).
2. The available resources.
3. The patient's (informed) values.
4. The research knowledge ('know–what' knowledge).

Poor decision making in nursing usually happens when nurses use the wrong type of information to inform their decisions or place too much emphasis on a particular form of information (Dowding and Thompson, 2004). Therefore, it is crucial to ensure that when making decisions the appropriate sources of information are accessed. When studying decision making in nurses, Rycroft-Malone et al. (2009) found that nurses used a range of strategies, drawing on informal protocols – local ways of working – interactions with co-workers and patients, instinct and formal protocols. However, the primary approach used was interactions with others: here, nurses discussed decisions made with colleagues and preferred to approach more senior colleagues for information rather than turning to protocols. Protocol-based care has generally been advocated as helping health professionals reach the 'best' decision in relation to the situation they seek to facilitate. It is said these simplify and aid decision making, promoting standardised practice based on best available evidence in the form of care pathways, guidelines and/or algorithms. Rycroft-Malone et al. (2009) found that less experienced staff tended to use protocols more frequently, but as individuals became more experienced there was a tendency to rely on memory and past experiences. Although nurses recognised that protocols should be used more frequently, time constraints were said to reduce ability to refer to these. Protocols were often referred to after delivering care to see if decisions made fell within stated guidelines. Nurses expressed a belief that protocols encouraged standardisation, which it was felt did not necessarily equate to best practice as it was seen as being impersonal and, therefore, challenged individualisation of care.

There are many different types of clinical decisions which nurses are called upon to make. Thompson et al. (2004) identified 11 different forms of decisions made in everyday practice (see Table 4.2).

Table 4.2   Forms of decisions made in practice

Intervention	Targeting	Timing	Prevention
Referral	Communication	Assessment	Diagnosis
Information	Experience	Service delivery	

Activity 4.6

Reflect on one recent day in clinical practice and consider if, when and how you were involved in the 11 types of decisions identified in Table 4.2. Identify how these decisions were made and whether you felt you had the appropriate evidence on which to base those decisions.

There are various conceptual models available to explain the factors involved in making a clinical decision. Tanner (2006) proposed that it is a four-stage process involving noticing, interpreting, responding and reflecting. Lasater (2007) identifies that each of these stages has specific components:

1. Noticing – observing, noticing change and collecting information.
2. Interpreting – making sense of the information and prioritising.
3. Responding – planning intervention, using clear communication and appropriate skills.
4. Reflecting – evaluating the incident and looking for ways to improve performance.

Standing (2017) suggested that clinical decision-making skills have 12 facets (see Table 4.3).

Table 4.3   Clinical decision-making skills

Collaboration	Experience and intuition	Confidence	Prevention
Systematic	Prioritising	Observation	Diagnosis
Standardisation	Reflectivity	Ethical sensitivity	Accountability

> Identify one patient whose care you were recently involved with. Consider each of Standing's decision-making skills and identify whether or not you used these in making care delivery decisions.

Activity 4.7

In making a clinical decision, it is proposed that a nurse's judgement is helped if the most up to date evidence is available and the needs of the service user are clearly identified. However, simply providing nurses with appropriate evidence will not in itself enhance the decision-making processes. Thompson (2003) put forward the notion of 'clinical uncertainty' in relation to decision making; that is, the idea that the practice of nursing takes place in the face of ever-changing demands. A patient's needs and status will change over time, thus resulting in complex and often competing demands.

If decision making is to be effective, then health professionals need to be aware of such changes and factor them into any decisions to be made. Therefore, it is necessary to consider the implications of a decision over time, what Melnyk and Fineout-Overholt (2018) describe as 'clinical forethought'. This has four components – future think, forethought about specific populations, anticipation of risks and the unexpected (see Table 4.4 for an overview). Issues that may have an impact on, and implications for, care delivery should be identified and considered. Clinical judgement is used in managing these uncertainties and arriving at a decision as to how to proceed – many see this as the 'art' of nursing – and is central to clinical expertise.

Table 4.4   Clinical forethought

Type	Description
Future think	Considering the immediate future and anticipating issues that might arise
	Identifying immediate resources needed
	Considering future responses
	Evaluating judgement and making adjustments as necessary

(Continued)

Table 4.4   (Continued)

Type	Description
Specific patients	Considering general trends in patient experiences and responses to intervention
	Identifying local resources available to deal with potential issues
Risks	Anticipating particular issues that may impact on a specific individual – such as anxiety, distress
The unexpected	Expecting the unexpected
	Anticipating the need to respond to new situations and resources – yours and organisational – if difficulties arise

Activity 4.8

Imagine you are about to administer a new form of medication to a patient for the first time. What 'clinical forethought' issues can you identify?

As identified above, nurses' personal knowledge and experience have the greatest impact on these decision–making activities, moulding how the nurse interprets the situation and deals with the uncertainties. The greater the knowledge/experience, the larger the number of perspectives and possibilities that are likely to be identified. As discussed in Chapter 2, Benner (1984) proposed that the 'expert' nurse draws on knowledge in an intuitive way and reaches conclusions without being able to verbalise the process by which those decisions were reached (see Chapter 2 in relation to tacit knowledge). However, Fitzpatrick (2007) suggested an expert nurse in relation to EBP needs to be able to make clear and reasoned links between theory and practice with the ability to integrate patient perspectives into this 'mix'.

Nursing expertise is defined by Higgs and Titchen (2001: 274) as the 'professional artistry and practice wisdom inherent in professional practice'. Clinical expertise is viewed by Manley et al. (2005) as having a number of components (see Box 4.1). The development of these aspects of clinical expertise are said to be linked to 'enabling factors' – the ability to reflect; to organise practice giving consideration to overarching influences; to work autonomously; to develop good interpersonal relationships; and to promote respect.

Box 4.1   Nursing expertise

1. Holistic practice knowledge – integrating various forms of knowledge, academic and experiential, into their delivery of care.

2. Knowing the patient – respecting the patient's views/perspectives, encouraging patient decision making and promoting independence.
3. Moral agency promoting respect, dignity and self-efficacy in others whilst maintaining one's own professional integrity.
4. Saliency – observing and picking up on cues from patients, recognising the needs of patients and others.
5. Skilled know-how – problem solving, responding to the changing environment of care and adapting to needs as appropriate.
6. Change catalyst – promoting appropriate change.
7. Risk taker – weighing the risks and taking appropriate decisions, to achieve best patient outcomes.

APPROACHES TO DECISION MAKING

There are a number of frameworks that can be used to help with decision making.

Facione and Gittens (2013: 47) offered a five-step approach to effective thinking and problem solving known as IDEAS:

I = IDENTIFY the Problem and Set Priorities (Step 1)

D = DEEPEN Understanding and Gather Relevant Information (Step 2)

E = ENUMERATE Options and Anticipate Consequences (Step 3)

A = ASSESS the Situation and Make a Preliminary Decision (Step 4)

S = SCRUTINISE the Process and Self-Correct as Needed (Step 5)

Consider an area of concern in your area of practice. Using Facione and Gittens' framework, identify how best to address the issues of concern.

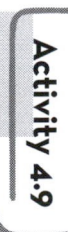

Activity 4.9

Hoffman et al. (2010) proposed a clinical reasoning cycle, based on research concerning expert nurses' thought and decision-making processes. It was suggested that this cycle can be used to promote the development of practice-specific knowledge and clinical reasoning skills in students and novice practitioners. There are eight steps in the cycle:

1. Describe the patient and the context of their care situation.
2. Consider all the information currently available (notes, charts, history) and gather any further information needed. Apply the theoretical knowledge you already have to the patient's illness/presentation and the situation.

3. Review all the data you have to get a full picture of the patient and their context. Identify what is and is not relevant, and any patterns and relationships between the various pieces of information. Compare the current situation to your past experiences and suggest possible outcomes.
4. Evaluate the information to clarify the nature of the problem to be addressed.
5. Set your goals and time frame within which these will be achieved.
6. Implement your plan of action.
7. Evaluate outcomes.
8. Reflect on the experience and identify learning needs.

Activity 4.10

When in your own area of practice use Hoffman et al.'s framework in relation to a specific patient problem.

Carroll and Johnson (1990) suggested an alternative seven-stage model of decision making, which does not follow a linear pattern but can be repeated or returned to as necessary:

1. Recognition of the situation.
2. Formulation of explanation.
3. Alternative generation of other explanations.
4. Information search to clarify choices and available evidence.
5. Judgement or choice.
6. Action.
7. Feedback.

Activity 4.11

Think about the above three frameworks and decide which one reflects your decision-making process in clinical practice.

EBP calls for a more analytical approach to making clinical decisions, and it is anticipated there will be a conscious weighing up of the options and consideration of the various issues. The McMaster's EBM group caution against the use of clinical experience and intuition in the absence of evidence based on systematic observation in making clinical judgements (Eraut, 2000). However, it should not be underestimated how much interpretation may be needed in deciding how evidence should be used – EBP cannot always provide concrete evidence on which to base practice. A possible model for this process is given in Figure 4.2.

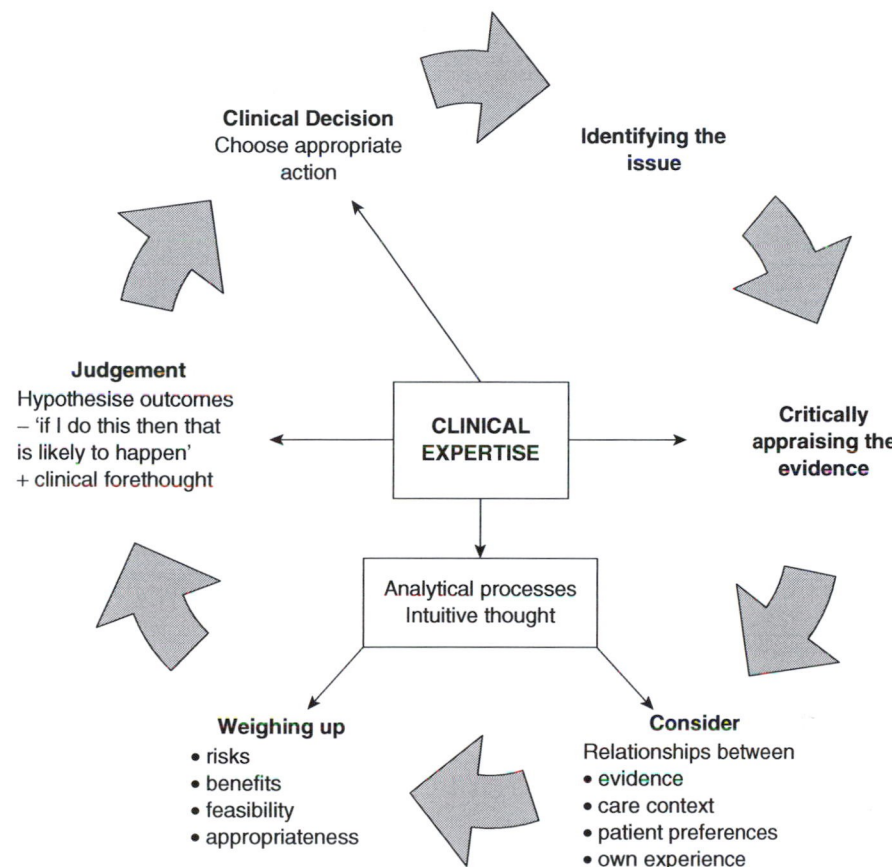

Figure 4.2   Model for clinical decision making

GROUP DECISION MAKING

Healthcare does not take place in a vacuum but is delivered by a team of professionals and ancillary staff. Many of the decisions made in clinical practice are taken collectively. This brings both advantages and disadvantages. By definition, group decisions are participatory and subject to social influence. Perhaps the greatest advantage is that group members tend to be from different specialties and as such provide more information and knowledge. Implementation of the decision is more effective since the people who are putting the decision into practice have contributed to its formulation and feel an investment in it. The participative nature of group decision making means that it can act as a training ground for junior members of staff to develop the skills of questioning and objective analysis and for senior members of staff to act as role-models. The seven-step model presented below offers a structured approach to group decision making.

1. Identify the decision to be made.
2. Examine the data. Perhaps most importantly ask what additional information is needed.
3. Establish criteria. Identify the criteria or conditions that would determine whether a chosen solution is successful.
4. Discuss potential solutions based on the available evidence.
5. Evaluate options and select the best one. Remember not everyone will necessarily agree; however, whatever decision is reached should be based on the best evidence at the time.
6. Implement the solution.
7. Monitor and evaluate the outcome. (Adapted from University of Waterloo (2015))

Group decisions can also be less efficient that those made by an individual. Group decisions can take longer to reach and there may be conflict between group members as to what to do and what is the best evidence to support a particular approach. One of the biggest disadvantages to such decision making is the phenomenon known as Groupthink. Groupthink was a term first put forward by Irving Jarvis (1972) to describe the situation in which a group makes faulty decisions because group pressures lead to a deterioration of 'mental efficiency, reality testing and moral judgement' (1972: 9). Groupthink occurs when individuals in a group feel under pressure to conform to what seems to be the dominant view of the group, and can lead to the following barriers:

- incomplete survey of alternatives;
- incomplete survey of objectives;
- failure to examine risks of preferred choice;
- failure to reappraise initially rejected alternatives;
- poor information search;
- selective bias in processing information at hand;
- failure to work out contingency plans;
- low probability of successful outcome.

Activity 4.12

Ferguson and Day (2007) proposed that novice nurses lack confidence in their own clinical judgement and decision-making processes. Complete a SWOT analysis (see Appendix 1) in relation to your own skills in this area and identify your future learning needs.

Summary

- The complexity of care requires finely honed clinical judgement skills to ensure clinical decision making is of the highest standard.
- Nurses' experiences and perspectives/values have a greater impact on their clinical judgement than scientific evidence.
- Clinical judgement and clinical decision making are closely linked but separate concepts.
- Involvement of service users in the decisions and sound clinical decision making are central to EBP.
- Clinical judgement is seen as the 'art' of nursing and central to clinical expertise, and involves the weighing up of options and reaching a decision as to appropriate action.
- Both analytical process and intuitive thinking are central to clinical judgement.

FURTHER READING

Standing, M. (2017) *Clinical Judgement and Decision Making in Nursing* (3rd edn) Transforming Nursing Practice Series. London: Sage. This provides an in-depth exploration of issues related to clinical judgement and decision making.

USEFUL WEBLINKS

NHS National Prescribing Centre: has a series of short videos related to EBP and decision making, including individual decision making. www.npc.nhs.uk/evidence/making_decisions_better/making_decisions_better.php

5

Finding the Evidence
Marishona Ortega and Janet Barker

Learning Outcomes

By the end of the chapter you will be able to:

- identify and choose appropriate resources when finding evidence;
- understand the use of keywords, subject headings and other techniques when searching for evidence;
- develop a search strategy to locate relevant literature.

INTRODUCTION

It is important that all nurses and other healthcare professionals develop the skills of being able to find, interpret and use up to date evidence as it is integral to evidence-based practice, which has been defined as 'the integration of the best research evidence with our clinical expertise and our patient's unique values and circumstances' (Straus et al., 2019).

Searching for 'best research evidence' is an important skill to develop and, as Greenhalgh (2014) has pointed out, you may be rigorous in critically appraising the evidence but if you are considering the wrong paper then this is a waste of your time and effort. Most forms of evidence are now available online so an important part of finding evidence is being able to navigate your way through the myriad of resources available. This chapter will introduce you to some of the key aspects related to identifying and choosing appropriate sources of evidence.

WHERE IS THE EVIDENCE?

Evidence can take many forms and this chapter will look at different types of evidence both published and unpublished. The value and credibility of each type must be considered when trying to establish if it is going to be useful to you and your professional practice.

Books

Books are often the starting point for many people in their search for evidence and they can offer:

- a general overview on a subject and help you identify key topics that you should be aware of;
- useful background information;
- a comparison of different theories;
- references to other sources of information, which you can follow up.

Books, however, will not be the place to find the latest thinking or research on a topic as the information you find in books can sometimes become dated due to the length of the publishing process. This is when you will need to use journals.

Journals

Journals are a primary means of communicating scholarly activity and provide a range of articles, from editorials and discussion pieces to case studies and clinical trials, all of which contribute to the evidence base, and are published at regular intervals, such as monthly or quarterly.

Discussion and commentary papers can also be important when considering concepts and theories that are central to a profession's knowledge base or where little is known about a topic. There are many thousands of journals in healthcare, and the information found within them will tend to be more specialised and up to date than that found in books.

Many journals provide alerting services, so that you can be informed when new issues come out and thus keep up to date with the latest thinking in your field.

Find out which journals in your subject area you can access via your health library.
Check whether you can access them in print or online.

Activity 5.1

Government and policy documents

Government and policy documents can prove a valuable source of information. Most of these can be found via the UK Government's website at www.gov.uk or via individual department sites, e.g. the Department of Health & Social Care at: www.gov.uk/government/organisations/department-of-health-and-social-care.

Repositories

Many universities and research institutes make their research outputs available in an institutional repository, which can hold a wide range of material including preliminary versions of journal articles, data sets, interview records, etc. OpenDOAR (http://v2.sherpa.ac.uk/opendoar/) is the quality-assured global directory of academic open access repositories, which allows you to search both for repositories and their contents.

Research in progress

It is also possible to find out about research in progress or the very latest research findings on the following sites:

- National Institute for Health Research (NIHR)'s Dissemination Centre critically appraises the latest health research to identify and make public the most significant findings. Available at: www.ukctg.nihr.ac.uk/clinical-trials/latest-research-findings
- UK Clinical Trials Gateway. Find clinical trials by condition or geographical location. Available at: www.ukctg.nihr.ac.uk
- PROSPERO, an international register of prospectively registered systematic reviews in health and social care. Available at: www.crd.york.ac.uk/PROSPERO/
- EU Clinical Trials Register contains information on clinical trials conducted in the European Union (EU), or the European Economic Area (EEA), which started after May 2004. Available at: www.clinicaltrialsregister.eu
- The World Health Organization's International Clinical Trials Registry Platform provides access to a central database containing the trial registration data sets from a range of providers from around the world. It also provides links to the full original records. Available at: http://apps.who.int/trialsearch
- The US National Library of Medicine maintains clinicaltrials.gov, which includes trials and interventional studies from over 200 countries. Available at: http://clinicaltrials.gov

Grey literature

Another important source of evidence is known as **grey literature**. This is literature that has not been formally published, but nevertheless may include useful information. Grey literature can include:

Theses

There are several resources that can be searched for theses and/or dissertations, which are undertaken as part of a course of study for various levels of degree (masters and doctorates):

- EThOS – the UK's national thesis service provided by the British Library holds records of nearly 500,000 theses awarded by over 120 institutions. Available at: http://ethos.bl.uk
- DART-Europe e-theses provides a single European portal for the discovery of electronic theses and dissertations. Available at: www.dart-europe.eu

- Open Access Dissertation & Theses from over 1,100 colleges, universities and research institutions. Available at: https://oatd.org
- Proquest Dissertations & Theses Global is a single repository of graduate dissertations and theses from universities in 88 countries (subscription required)

In-house publications

In-house publications, for example, leaflets, pamphlets, newsletters and reports. The internet is often a good source for locating these. However, there are some specialist databases that include:

- HMIC (Health Management and Information Consortium) includes publications from the Department of Health and The King's Fund (subscription required)
- Open Grey is a multidisciplinary European database, covering science, technology, biomedical science, economics, social science and humanities. Available at: www.opengrey.eu

Conferences

Conference papers and presentations can give you an insight into the cutting edge of research where new theories may be presented before they are published in a journal article; however, they can sometimes be difficult to locate. Some conference papers may be included in subject-specific databases such as Medline or CINAHL, but there are additional resources available:

- Conference Proceedings Citation Index via Web of Science includes global coverage of nearly 150,000 conferences (subscription required)
- ZeTOC, produced by the British Library allows you to search for conference papers and set up alerts. Available at: http://zetoc.jisc.ac.uk/ (subscription required)
- Over 7 million conference papers from proceedings and journals are indexed on Scopus (subscription required)
- Google Scholar includes conferences from specific publishers. Available at: https://scholar.google.co.uk

Searching the internet

Search engines are designed to find information on the internet and Google is the most popular and well known. Tempting as it may be to search for all your evidence on Google, be aware that not all websites are suitable for finding evidence on which to base your practice. Some information that you find will be well researched and well written, but you may also come across information that is at best misleading, at worst, incorrect. Evidence-based practice is about finding the 'best research evidence' and Google may not help you do this, as there are several potential issues that you need to be aware of:

- It is not sufficiently focused to meet all your needs when looking for evidence. For example, at the time of writing, a search for 'smoking and hypnotherapy' on Google produced 2.8 million results. It would be an immense task to look at every result and would not be good use of your time as you may find yourself looking at lots of irrelevant information.

- Anyone can publish information on the internet; information you find may be based on insubstantial evidence or may be biased in that it only presents one point of view. You need to have the skills to be able to filter the good sites from the bad.
- Information can be out–of–date.
- You may miss out on finding the latest research as this information may only be available from specialist websites or databases that require a subscription.

It is essential that you do not rely solely on general search engines such as Google and that you instead familiarise yourself with, and use, those that are specifically aimed at nurses and other healthcare professions. See Box 5.1 for examples of suggested search engines.

Box 5.1   Suggested search engines

1. Google Scholar: searches a broad range of scholarly literature. Available at: https://scholar.google.co.uk
2. NICE Evidence: a unique source of authoritative, evidence-based information from hundreds of trustworthy and accredited sources. Includes access to journals and databases (requires an NHS OpenAthens account). Available at: www.evidence.nhs.uk
3. SUMSearch 2: simultaneously searches for original studies, systematic reviews, and practice guidelines from PubMed. Available at: http://sumsearch.org
4. TRIP: a clinical search engine containing high-quality evidence-based health information to support practice and/or care. Available at: www.tripdatabase.com

---

Activity 5.2

Choose and locate one of the search engines identified in Box 5.1. Search for an area of practice that you would like to know more about. How many 'hits' are identified? Consider whether the results are sufficiently focused to meet your needs in searching for evidence.

WHAT RESOURCES ARE AVAILABLE TO HELP WITH EBP?

With the explosion of information and knowledge available on which to base practice, busy practitioners can find themselves overwhelmed. For example, the database MEDLINE contains over 25 million citations with over 800,000 records added in 2017 alone (US National Library of Medicine, 2018). There is also a need to ensure that you find the best evidence in relation to your area of interest – not all literature is good evidence and you need to learn to identify the strengths, limitations and applicability to your question of any evidence you find, which is where the skills of critical appraisal are required (see Part II of this book). Over the last two decades, various hierarchies of pre-appraised evidence have been developed and have evolved as new resources and services become available. The most recent iteration is Alper and Haynes' (2016) Evidence-based Healthcare (EHBC) Pyramid 5.0, where five categories of resources have been identified and prioritised to help practitioners find appropriate evidence to use when making decisions about care delivery. Starting at the top of the hierarchy, the five levels are:

1. Systems
2. Synthesised summaries for clinical reference
3. Systematically derived recommendations (guidelines)
4. Systematic reviews
5. Studies

Each level builds systematically on information from the lower levels to 'provide substantially more useful information for guiding clinical decision-making' (Alper and Haynes, 2016).

Systems are describes as computerised decision support systems (CDSSs) which can integrate and summarise all available and appropriate evidence related to a particular clinical issue, and when linked to a specific patient's circumstances (electronic health record), propose appropriate action. These systems integrate and summarise all available and appropriate evidence related to a specific clinical issue, and when linked to an individual patient's circumstances (electronic health record), propose appropriate action. According to Windish (2013), these systems are still evolving and are not currently widespread. Therefore, if a system is not available, the next level down the hierarchy is to look for **synthesised summaries for clinical reference**, which integrate the three lower layers of the hierarchy and include online clinical textbooks. These texts provide an evidence-based summary of best practice at the point of care, which are regularly updated.

Examples include:

- UptoDate – www.uptodate.com
- Dynamed Plus – https://dynamed.ebscohost.com
- BMJ Best Practice – https://bestpractice.bmj.com/info
- Essential Evidence Plus – www.essentialevidenceplus.com

Systematically derived recommendations (guidelines) are similar to synthesised summaries but will generally focus on a single condition or disease such as the assessment and management of bipolar disorder.

Providers include:

- National Institute for Health & Care Excellence (NICE) guidelines. Available at: www.nice.org.uk

- Scottish Intercollegiate Guidelines Network (SIGN) guidelines. Available at: www.sign.ac.uk
- Profession-specific guidance produced by organisations or charities

Systematic reviews provide rigorous reviews of evidence relating to specific areas of interest and are also advocated as high-quality sources of information. Individual reviews can be found in several resources including:

- Cochrane Database of Systematic Reviews, which focuses on the effectiveness of healthcare interventions. Available at: www.cochranelibrary.com
- Campbell Library of Systematic Reviews, which focuses on the effects of social interventions in crime and justice, education and social welfare. Available at: https://campbell collaboration.org/library
- Joanna Briggs Institute's Database of Systematic Reviews and Implementation Reports. Available at: https://journals.lww.com/jbisrir

Alper and Haynes also suggest that guidelines, systematic reviews and studies should be subdivided into filtered (pre-appraised) and synopses (appraised and extracted), which means that you don't need to assess the quality yourself. The following resources may also prove useful:

- EvidenceAlerts – a key source of pre-appraised synthese – https://plus.mcmaster.ca/evidencealerts/Default.aspx
- Evidence-based abstraction journals such as:
    - *Evidence-Based Nursing* – http://ebn.bmj.com
    - *Evidence-Based Mental Health* – http://ebmh.bmj.com
    - *Evidence-Based Medicine* – https://ebm.bmj.com
    - *ACP Journal Club* – http://annals.org/aim/journal-club

However, if your area of interest is not covered by any of the resources listed above, then your ultimate source will be original **studies**, which you will need to appraise to identify their strengths, limitations and applicability to your question. This is where you will need to develop your skills in searching for evidence.

SEARCHING FOR EVIDENCE

Searching for evidence or literature searching is a skill that takes time and practice to develop. Many of the resources discussed below will have online tutorials that guide you through the steps you need to take to make best use of them and it is well worth spending some time working through these. Your health librarian will also be able to help you develop the skills that you need, so it is advisable to book an appointment to see them individually or attend a training session. It will be time well spent and save you a great deal of effort and frustration later when you are searching for evidence to support your practice.

There are a number of steps to follow when searching for evidence:

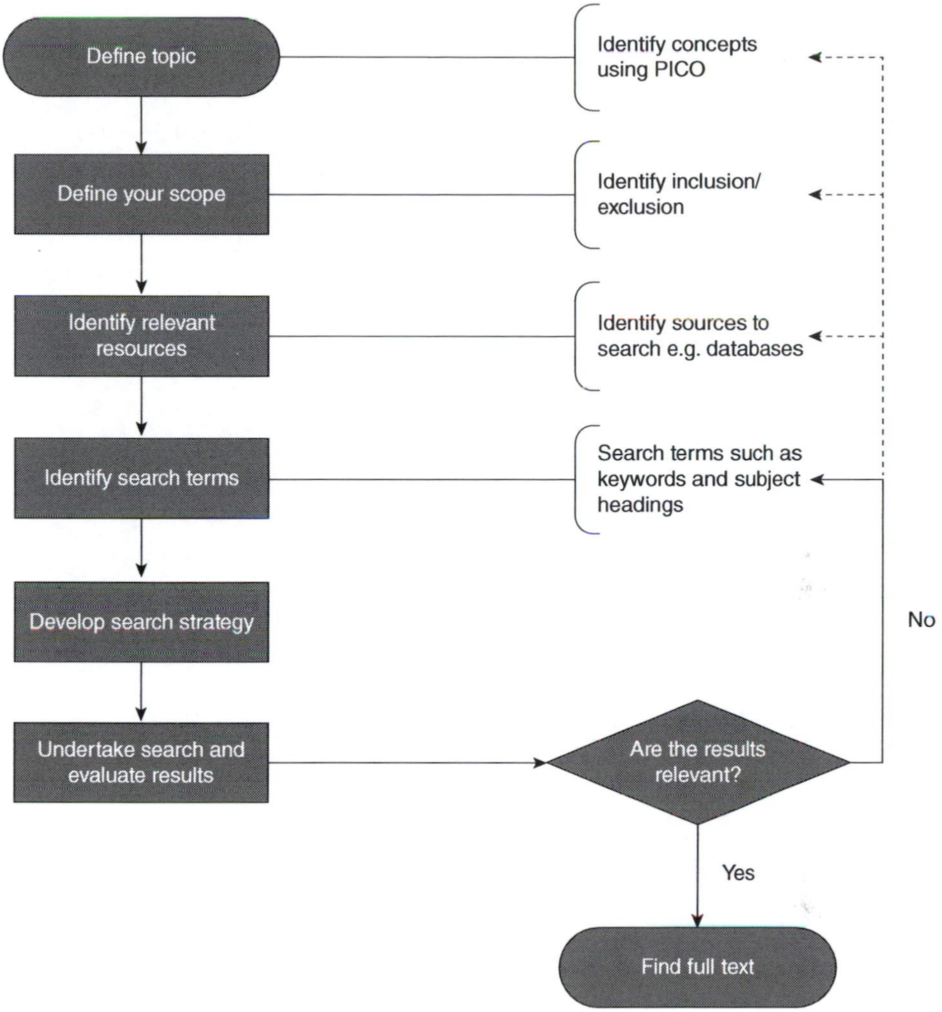

Figure 5.1   Flowchart showing the steps of searching for evidence

Define your topic

Although it is tempting to start searching straightaway, it is a good idea to plan your search by defining your topic. This will ensure that your search has a focus, which should mean that you do not retrieve lots of irrelevant results.

As discussed in Chapter 2, a good way to structure your search is to use the PICO model, which is ideal for clinical questions where a healthcare intervention is involved (Richardson et al., 1995). The terms you identify using PICO will form the main concepts of your search strategy and will help you focus on what you are looking for.

P = Patient, problem or population – who are the people that you are interested in? Do they have similar characteristics, i.e. gender, age, ethnicity or disease/condition?

I = Intervention – how are you considering intervening – drugs, surgery, etc.?

C = Comparison – is there an alternative that you wish to compare? This could be comparing two different types of interventions or comparing an intervention against no intervention

O = Outcome – what is the effect of the intervention? This could be a reduction in symptoms, benefits or improved prognosis, e.g. smoking cessation

For example, if PICO was applied to the question 'What is the effectiveness of hypnotherapy compared to nicotine replacement therapy for helping people to quit smoking?' it would look like Table 5.1.

Table 5.1   Main concepts of a search strategy using PICO

Patient/problem	Intervention	Comparison	Outcome
Smokers	Hypnotherapy	Nicotine Replacement Therapy	Smoking cessation

There are alternative frameworks for literature searching available, including:

* PICOC – **P**opulation, **I**ntervention, **C**omparison, **O**utcome, **C**ontext (Petticrew and Roberts, 2006);
* ECLIPSE – **E**xpectation, **C**lient group, **L**ocation, **I**mpact, **P**rofessionals, **S**ervice – useful for health policy/management topics (Wildridge and Bell, 2002);
* SPICE – **S**etting, **P**erspective, **I**ntervention, **C**omparison, **E**valuation – useful for qualitative studies or the social sciences (Booth, 2004);
* SPIDER – **S**ample, **P**henomenon of Interest, **D**esign, **E**valuation, **R**esearch type – useful for qualitative and mixed methods studies (Cooke et al., 2012).

Activity 5.3

Select an area that you would like to know more about and identify the Patient/problem, Intervention, Comparison and Outcome (PICO) using the form in Appendix 3.

Define your scope

It is also a good idea to define the scope of your search. This is where you consider any *inclusion or exclusion criteria*, which will help to focus your search and increase the likelihood of retrieving relevant literature.

Examples of inclusion criteria:

- Literature published in the English language
- Literature published since 2015
- Randomised controlled trials (RCTs) only

Examples of exclusion criteria:

- Literature published in a non-English language
- Literature published before 2015
- Non-randomised controlled trials (Non-RCTs)

Define the scope of your PICO question in Appendix 3 – do you want to limit your search in any way?

Activity 5.4

Identify relevant resources to search

To ensure that you are aware of what is available on a given topic and access the most up to date information, you will need to search databases. Databases contain records of journal articles, dissertations, book chapters, reviews, etc. often in a specific subject area. They enable users to search for information by keyword, subject headings and descriptors, and will sometimes provide full-text access to the journal articles in question.

The databases that are of interest here are those related to the healthcare professions, and some suggested databases are listed in Box 5.2. The ones most commonly used by nurses and healthcare professionals are CINAHL (Cumulative Index to Nursing and Allied Health Literature) and MEDLINE. CINAHL is one of the most comprehensive databases for nurses and allied health professions. It has over 3.8 million records from 3,100 plus journals and covers many English-language journals (EBSCO, 2018). It also indexes some books, book chapters and nursing dissertations. There are various versions of CINAHL, including CINAHL Complete, which provides full-text access to 1,300 journals. Access is via subscription only and therefore it will depend upon what your library subscribes to as to what will be available to you.

MEDLINE is produced by the United States National Library of Medicine and contains more than 25 million citations from over 5,200 journals (US National Library of Medicine, 2018). Although the majority of journals indexed are medical, it also indexes a number of nursing journals. There are various online versions of MEDLINE and it can be freely accessed using PubMed.

There are a number of information service providers, through which education and health communities can access a range of databases and support services from one platform. Examples include Ovid and EBSCOhost and NICE's HDAS (Healthcare Databases Advanced Search). Many service providers (e.g. HDAS) allow you to search across multiple databases, which will help save you time and effort.

The search interfaces may differ slightly, but the principles of searching will be the same. Most will offer both basic and advanced searching as well as allowing you to combine and save searches. However, the easiest way to learn how to get the most out of searching the databases available to you is by booking a training session with your health librarian or by working through the online tutorials for each database.

Box 5.2   Suggested databases

AMED: allied and complementary medicine database. Includes citations from over 600 journals related to allied health professions, complementary medicine and palliative care (subscription required).

BNI (British Nursing Index): UK nursing and midwifery database of over 700 journals (subscription required).

CINAHL (Cumulative Index to Nursing and Allied Health Literature): literature relating to nursing and allied health professions from over 3,100 journals (subscription required).

Cochrane Library: a collection of six databases providing high-quality evidence to inform decision making. This includes the Cochrane Database of Systematic Reviews, which contains full-text systematic reviews providing an overview of the effects of interventions on healthcare and Cochrane Protocols, which provide information about reviews in progress. Available at: www.cochranelibrary.com.

EMBASE (Excerpta Medica): an international biomedical database, similar to MEDLINE but having a greater focus on drugs and pharmacology (subscription required).

MEDLINE: the primary source for biomedical data from 1966 to the present. Compiled by the US National Library of Medicine (subscription required).

MIDIRS Reference Database: over 400 journals and other resources related to midwifery (subscription required).

PEDro (Physiotherapy Evidence Database): a free database of over 40,000 randomised trials, systematic reviews and clinical practice guidelines in physiotherapy. Available at: https://pedro.org.au

OTSeeker: a database that contains abstracts of systematic reviews, randomised controlled trials and other resources relevant to occupational therapy interventions. Please note that due to a lack of funding, content from 2016 onwards is not comprehensive. Available at: www.otseeker.com

PsycINFO: is the largest resource devoted to peer-reviewed literature in mental health and behavioural sciences. Compiled by the American Psychological Association it includes journal articles, books, book chapters and dissertations (subscription required).

PubMed: provides free web access to MEDLINE and contains more than 28 million records for biomedical literature, life science journals and online books. Records may include links to full-text content from PubMed Central or publisher websites. Available at: www.ncbi.nlm.nih.gov/pubmed

ScienceDirect: access to 3,800 journals and over 37,000 books from the scientific, technical and health disciplines (subscription required).

Social Care Online: a free database provided by the Social Care Institute for Excellence (SCIE). Includes legislation, government documents, practice and guidance, systematic reviews, research briefings, reports, journal articles and websites. Available at: www.scie-socialcareonline.org.uk

SCOPUS: the largest abstract and citation database of peer-reviewed literature: scientific journals, books and conference proceedings. Contains over 71 million records from over 23,000 journals (subscription required).

Web of Science/Knowledge: a collection of databases in the fields of science, social sciences, arts and humanities. Includes conference proceedings (subscription required).

Find out which databases you can access via your library.
Look at your completed PICO question in Appendix 3 and list which databases are relevant to your search.

Activity 5.5

Databases generally store publication information in the form of article title, author(s), journal title, year, volume, issue and page numbers. Many will include an abstract, which is a short summary of the content of the article. Reading the abstract as well as the title will help you determine whether the article will be relevant to you. Figure 5.2 is an example of a record from PubMed.

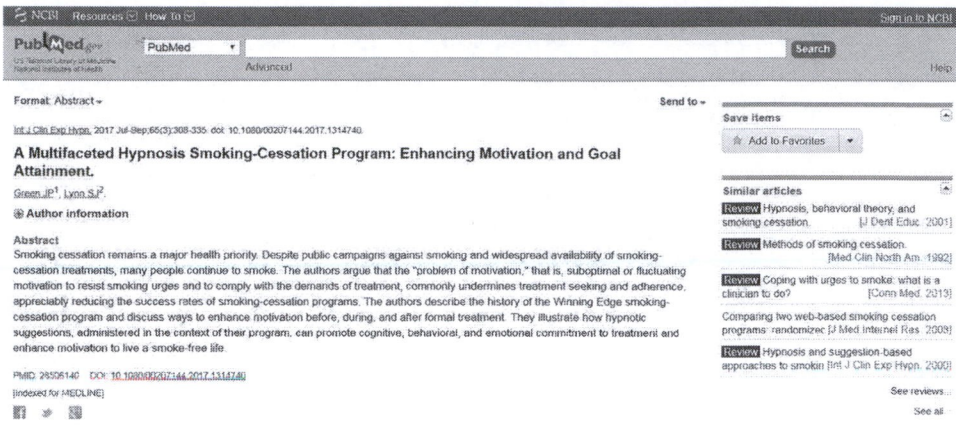

Figure 5.2   Example of a PubMed record

Available at: www.ncbi.nlm.nih.gov/pubmed/28506140 (accessed 20 July 2018).

Identify search terms

Having used PICO to identify the main concepts of your search, you should also consider and note:

- synonyms – words that share the same meaning (e.g. cancer and neoplasm);
- acronyms/abbreviations – where phrases have been shortened to a set of letters (e.g. CBT and cognitive behavioural therapy);
- alternative spellings (e.g. paediatrics and pediatrics);
- alternative terms (e.g. learning disabilities and learning disorders).

These will form the keywords that you will use in your search strategy.

Table 5.2 shows some possible alternative terms for our question: 'What is the effectiveness of hypnotherapy compared to nicotine replacement therapy for helping people to quit smoking?'

> **Activity 5.6**
>
> Look at the concepts you have identified in your PICO question in Appendix 3 and consider what other terms may be associated with them. You may have come up with a long list or just a few phrases. Whichever is the case, these are your keywords and will form part of your search strategy.

Develop a search strategy

A **search strategy** is the information (keywords, etc.) that you enter into the database to find the evidence that you want. These can be simple or complex – you will see in Chapter 9 that extensive searches are used in systematic reviews.

Table 5.2 Main concepts of a search strategy including a selection of alternative terms

Patient/problem	Intervention	Comparison	Outcome
Smoker	Hypnotherapy	Nicotine replacement	Smoking cessation
Smokers	Hypnosis	Nicotine replacement therapy	Tobacco use cessation
Smoking			Quit smoking
Tobacco use		NRT	
Cigarettes			

Boolean operators

These are the words '*and*', '*or*' and '*not*' which are used to combine search terms. For example, if you are interested in the effect hypnotherapy has on smoking, you may consider using the keywords smoking and hypnotherapy. A search of PubMed using the Boolean operators generated the following results:

Smoking *and* Hypnotherapy – 272 articles containing both words.

'*And*' narrows your search by only retrieving articles where both terms are present.

Smoking *or* Hypnotherapy – 270,201 articles containing either of the terms.

'*Or*' broadens your search by retrieving either term; this is useful where there are alternative terms for a concept that you wish to include in your strategy.

Smoking *not* Hypnotherapy – 255,513 articles containing Smoking but not Hypnotherapy.

'*Not*' should be used with caution in that you may exclude relevant articles that happen to mention the excluded term.

Table 5.3 includes Boolean operators to combine your search terms. This information can then be converted into your search strategy:

1. Smoker
2. Smokers
3. Smoking
4. Tobacco use
5. Cigarettes
6. 1 OR 2 OR 3 OR 4 OR 5
7. Hypnotherapy
8. Hypnosis
9. 7 OR 8

10. Nicotine replacement
11. Nicotine replacement therapy
12. NRT
13. 10 OR 11 OR 12
14. Smoking cessation
15. Tobacco use cessation
16. Quit smoking
17. 14 OR 15 OR 16
18. 6 AND 9 AND 13 AND 17

Table 5.3 Example of combining search terms using Boolean operators

Patient/ problem		Intervention		Comparison		Outcome
Smoker	**AND**	Hypnotherapy	**AND**	Nicotine replacement	**AND**	Smoking cessation
OR		**OR**		**OR**		**OR**
Smokers		Hypnosis		Nicotine replacement therapy		Tobacco use cessation
OR				**OR**		**OR**
Smoking				NRT		Quit smoking
OR						
Tobacco use						
OR						
Cigarettes						

Figure 5.3 shows what the strategy looks like in PubMed.

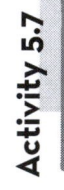

Activity 5.7 Type the keywords you identified earlier into a database of your choice and combine using Boolean operators. Note how many articles are retrieved.

Truncation

Truncation allows you to search for variations of words without having to include them all in your search strategy. A truncation mark (usually ★ or $ − check the database help guide

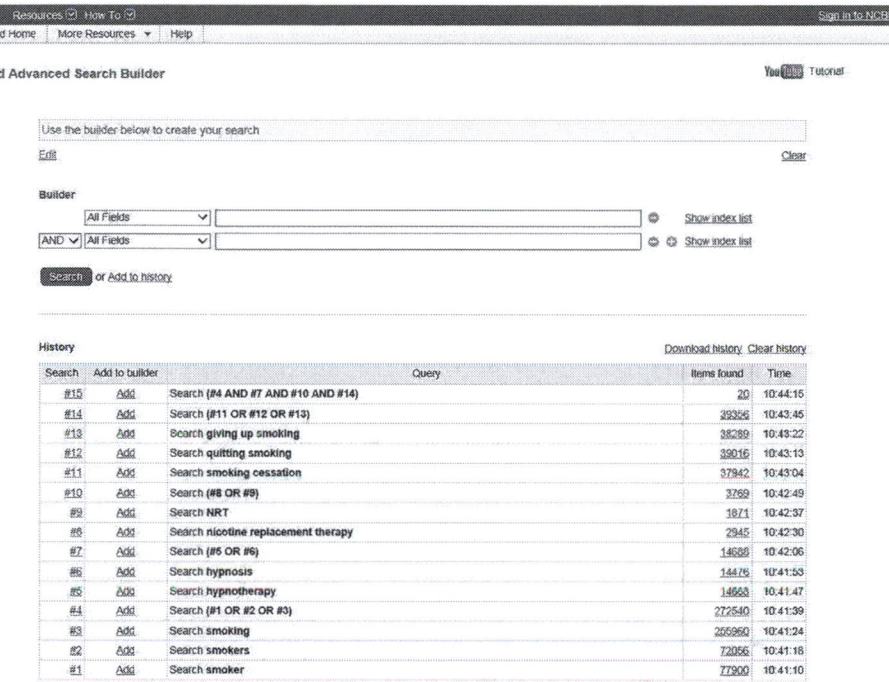

Figure 5.3 Example of a search using PubMed Advanced Search Builder using Boolean operators

Available at: www.ncbi.nlm.nih.gov/pubmed (accessed 20 July 2018)

as to which symbol should be used) put after a word–stem allows you to search for all the variations.

For example, PubMed uses ★ as truncation, so rather than searching for:

- Smoker
- Smokers
- Smoking

you could simply put smok★ and this will retrieve all the variations. This method can save you time when searching but it is important to be aware that this type of searching can generate lots of results as any passing reference to the word is retrieved. Consideration also needs to be given as to where to truncate words; for example, when searching PubMed for hypno★ over 45,000 records were retrieved, but in addition to articles about hypnotherapy or hypnosis, it also included articles about hypnotic drugs and hypnosedatives.

Phrase searching

In addition to searching for individual keywords, it is also possible to search for phrases by putting quotation marks (" ") around the terms, e.g. "nicotine replacement therapy", which means only records containing that exact phrase will be retrieved.

Wildcards

Where words may have alternative spellings – such as paediatrics and pediatrics – a symbol (often ? or # – check the database help guide as to which symbol should be used) can be placed within the word at the point where the variation may occur. In this example you would use "p?ediatrics" to ensure words with either the UK or American spelling will be then searched for and retrieved.

Adjacency operators

Many databases will allow you to search for a word within a specified number of another word of your choice. For example, in the EBSCOhost interface, "nicotine N2 replacement" will find the word nicotine within two words of replacement (regardless of the order in which they appear). These are called adjacency or proximity operators and they will generally differ between databases. Therefore, you should check the online help.

Field searching

One technique to increase the precision of your search is to restrict your search for keywords to specific fields of an article record, e.g. title or abstract. This means that results will only be retrieved where your specific keyword is in a specific field.

Subject headings

Many databases use a controlled vocabulary to describe and index the content of articles, with the most well known being Medical Subject Headings commonly known as MeSH, which is used in both MEDLINE and the Cochrane Library. CINAHL, for example, currently has over 15,000 subject headings (EBSCO Help, 2018), which are based on MeSH but with additional specific nursing and allied health headings added as appropriate. Subject headings are usually updated annually to reflect new developments.

Using subject headings combined with your keywords is a good way to ensure you are retrieving all relevant articles. Look for a link within the database that will take you to their subject headings, so that you can either browse or search them. MeSH is freely available to browse at: www.ncbi.nlm.nih.gov/mesh.

As can be seen in Figure 5.4, the recommended MeSH term for nicotine replacement products is "Tobacco Use Cessation Products". Subject headings can be included alongside your keywords in your search strategy.

An example of a search strategy using truncation, phrase searching and MeSH headings:

1. Smok★
2. Tobacco use
3. Cigarette★
4. Smoking [MeSH Terms]
5. Tobacco smoking [MeSH Terms]
6. 1 OR 2 OR 3 OR 4 OR 5

7. Hypnotherapy
8. Hypnosis
9. Hypnosis [MeSH Terms]
10. 7 OR 8 OR 9
11. "Nicotine replacement"
12. "Nicotine replacement therapy"
13. NRT
14. Tobacco Use Cessation Products [MeSH Terms]
15. 11 OR 12 OR 13 OR 14
16. "Smoking cessation"
17. "Tobacco use cessation"
18. "Quit smoking"
19. Smoking Cessation [MeSH Terms]
20. Tobacco Use Cessation [MeSH Terms]
21. 16 OR 17 OR 18 OR 19 OR 20
22. 6 AND 10 AND 15 AND 21

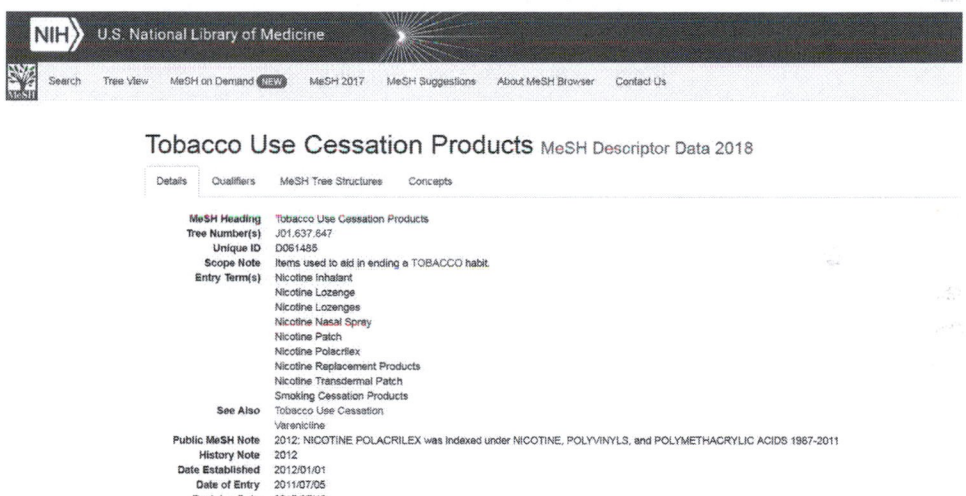

Figure 5.4   An extract for the entry in MeSH for tobacco use cessation products

Available at: meshb.nlm.nih.gov/record/ui?ui=D061485 (accessed 15 August 2018)

This strategy would retrieve articles potentially relevant to the original question "What is the effectiveness of hypnotherapy compared to nicotine replacement therapy for helping people to quit smoking?"

Figure 5.5 shows how the search strategy would look in PubMed.

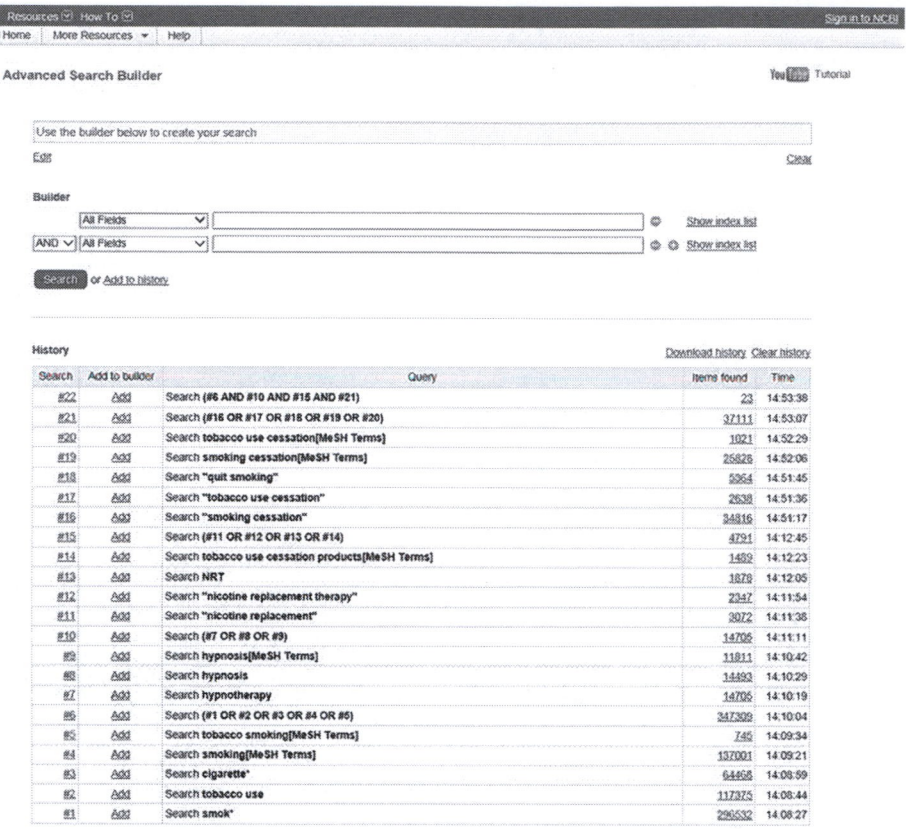

Figure 5.5   Example of a search using PubMed Advanced Search Builder using truncation, phrase searching and MeSH headings

Available at: www.ncbi.nlm.nih.gov/pubmed (accessed 9 August 2018)

Activity 5.8

Search the subject headings of your chosen database and check whether there are any associated with your keywords. Include these in your search strategy. Note how many articles are retrieved and compare this to your earlier search.

Limiting

Most databases allow you to limit your search in certain ways once your keywords and/or subject headings have been entered. This is where it is possible to limit your search according to your inclusion/exclusion criteria, which were identified as part of the planning process. For example, you may choose to limit by publication date – choosing a particular year or span of years. This can be useful if you are interested in the most recent information about a topic. Other limits include language – you may choose to retrieve only English-language articles; or patient group, which would include child, adult, etc. Some databases may allow you to limit your search to particular types of evidence – research papers, reviews, meta-analyses, etc.

Undertake search and evaluate results

It is important that when undertaking a search for evidence that you evaluate the results that are retrieved. You may not always be able to tell from an article title as to whether it is relevant to your question. Therefore, it is a good idea to also look at the abstract of the article, which will provide a short summary of the content. If you find that you have too many results, even after limiting your search by your inclusion criteria, then you may need to re-assess either your search strategy, the question that you are answering or both. Consider whether your search terms are too broad or whether the question is not focused enough.

Searching for evidence is an iterative process requiring continual review and refinement in order to develop an optimal search, which locates all relevant literature but ensures that you are not overwhelmed with irrelevant results.

Find full text

Once you have a list of results that are relevant to your question, the next step is to find the full text of the articles. Many databases will include links to the full text where it is available to you. If the full text is not available, remember that most libraries will offer an Inter-Library Loan or Document Supply service, whereby they are able to obtain journal articles (as well as books and other material) for you from other libraries, including the British Library. Contact your library for more details, including charges.

In recent years there has been a growth in "open access" publishing, where research findings are made freely available. Databases such as the Directory of Open Access Journals provide information from nearly 10,000 open access journals (available at: https://doaj.org).

ADDITIONAL SEARCHING TECHNIQUES

Citation pearl growing

Beyond browsing MeSH, there is an additional method of identifying search terms, known as **citation pearl growing**. This is where an article that exactly matches your criteria is located (the pearl) and it is then scanned to locate subject headings or other relevant key-words. These new terms can then be included in your search strategy.

Related articles

Many databases, including PubMed, provide links to "related articles", which will allow you to access articles on a similar subject. This can be useful in tracking down further relevant articles; however, it must be used with care as it is very easy to get side-tracked into areas that are related to, but not specifically, about your chosen topic.

Author searching

In addition to searching by keyword or subject heading, databases also give you the option of searching by authors' names. You may be aware that a particular author has written extensively on a topic. If so, you may want to search for literature written by that individual as this may lead you to other relevant articles.

Hand searching

You may find when looking through the results of your search that many relevant articles are published in one or two journals. Therefore, it may be useful to undertake a hand search of these journals, that is systematically (i.e. by hand) searching through each issue of the journal within your selected date range, to identify relevant literature. Although time-intensive, hand searching can be a useful technique to identify articles that have not been indexed correctly by a database.

Reference list searching

The reference lists of relevant articles can be scanned to identify other further articles of interest.

MANAGING YOUR REFERENCES

Most databases include the facility to save searches, save, print or email links to articles as well as export results to reference management software such as EndNote or RefWorks. This software can help you keep track of useful references as well as create reference lists or bibliographies in different referencing styles such as Harvard or Vancouver. If your library doesn't subscribe to this software, there are freely available tools such as Zotero (www.zotero.org) and Mendeley (www.mendeley.com) that you can use to manage and store your references.

STEPS TO SUCCESS

When searching for literature there are a few simple steps that will help you with the process:

- Find out what databases are available to you through your library.
- Familiarise yourself with the databases and how they work – what subject headings, truncation and wildcard symbols, etc. are used in each.
- When identifying your search terms be precise about what it is you want to find.

- Remember that your search terms can be combined using Boolean operators to build a search strategy.
- Limit your search as appropriate, e.g. by date, language or study type.
- Evaluate the results and refine your search as necessary.
- If you need help, remember your health librarian can assist you with finding the best available evidence.

Having completed the "Forming a Question and Searching for Evidence" template in Appendix 3 try out your search on one of the databases and evaluate the results. Reflect on your learning and identify areas where your searching skills need to improve.

Activity 5.9

Summary

- There are resources available to help you integrate evidence into practice – systems, synthesised summaries for clinical reference, systematically derived recommendations (guidelines) and systematic reviews.
- The key to finding evidence is having a clear and focused question. The PICO model can be used in this process.
- It is important to be aware of what resources are relevant to your subject and available to you when searching for evidence.
- Many databases use a controlled vocabulary (subject headings) to describe and index the content of articles, e.g. MeSH. Combining keywords with subject headings using Boolean operators can provide the means to locating relevant literature.
- Techniques such as using truncation or wildcards can help streamline your search.
- Searching for evidence is a skill that takes time and practice to develop and librarians are a key resource in helping you find the information that you need.

FURTHER READING

Aveyard, H. and Sharp, P. (2017) *A Beginner's Guide to Evidence Based Practice in Health and Social Care* (3rd edn). London: Open University Press/McGraw Hill Education.

Bettany-Saltikov, J. and McSherry, R. (2016) *How to Do a Systematic Literature Review in Nursing: A Step-By-Step Guide* (2nd edn). London: Open University Press/McGraw Hill Education.

Booth, A., Sutton, A. and Papaioannou, D. (2016) *Systematic Approaches to a Successful Literature Review* (2nd edn). London: Sage.

Czaplewski, L.M. (2012) 'Searching the literature: a researcher's perspective', *Journal of Infusion Nursing*, 35(1): 20–6.

Gerrish, K. and Lathlean, J. (eds) (2015) *The Research Process in Nursing* (7th edn). Oxford: Wiley Blackwell.

Greenhalgh, T. (2014) *How to Read a Paper: The Basics of Evidence-Based Medicine* (5th edn). Oxford: John Wiley & Sons/BMJ Books.

Jameson, J. and Walsh, M.E. (2017) 'Tools for evidence-based vascular nursing practice: achieving information literacy for lifelong learning', *Journal of Vascular Nursing*, 35(4): 201–10.

Moule, P., Aveyard, H. and Goodman, M. (2017) *Nursing Research: An Introduction* (3rd edn). London: Sage.

Stillwell, S.B., Fineout-Overholt, E., Melnyk, B.M. and Williamson, K.M. (2010) 'Evidence-based practice, step by step: searching for the evidence', *American Journal of Nursing*, 110(5): 41–7.

Conclusion to Part I

The aim of this section was to provide you with an underpinning knowledge of the various aspects of evidence-based practice and the skills associated with the first four aspects of the process as identified in Chapter 1. That is:

- the ability to identify what counts as appropriate evidence;
- forming a question to enable you to find evidence for consideration;
- developing a search strategy;
- finding the evidence.

This section ends with a crossword puzzle, with clues to answers relevant to Chapters 1, 2, 3, 4 and 5. The answers can be found on p. 222.

CROSSWORD PUZZLE

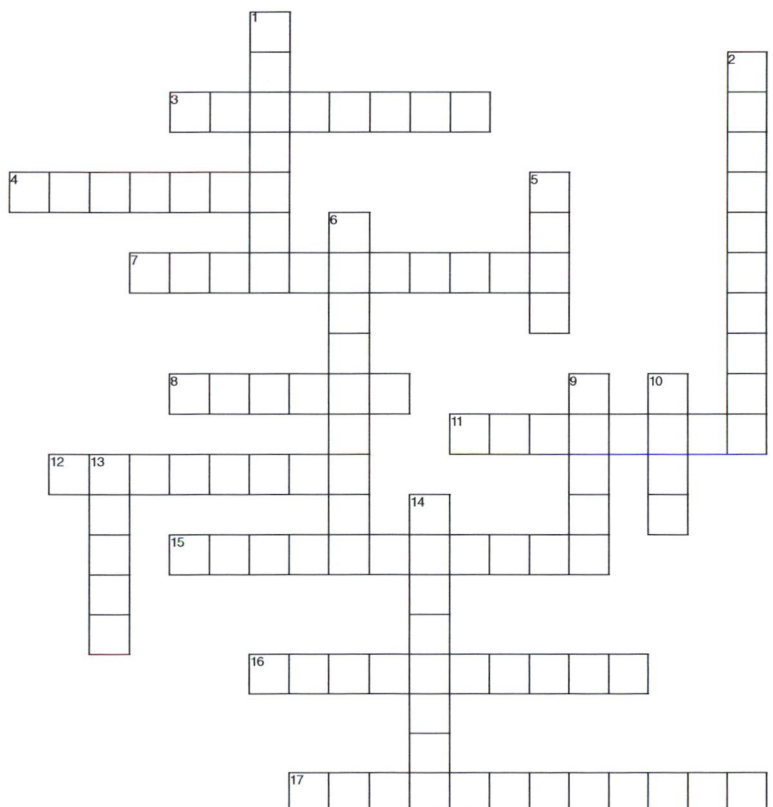

Across

3. Information on which to base best practice (8)
4. Words used to combine search terms (7)
7. Items of evidence grouped together to provide a greater effect (11)
8. Theorist's surname – proposed a framework of nursing knowledge (6)
11. Set of logically connected ideas (8)
12. Central point for storing information in relation to specific topics (8)
15. Considering implications of decisions over time (11)
16. Belief that only what can be observed can be called fact (10)
17. Belief that humans actively construct their reality (12)

Down

1. A body of knowledge organised in a systematic way (7)
2. The belief that reality is ordered and can be studied objectively (10)
5. Terms used to describe medical subject headings (4)
6. Essential aspect of clinical decision making (9)
9. Knowledge used by practitioners drawn from experience (5)
10. Format for creating search questions (4)
13. Process for gathering information to promote effective care (5)
14. Last name of the 'father' of EBM (8)

PART II
Critiquing the Evidence

6

What is Critical Appraisal?

Ros Kane and Janet Barker

Learning Outcomes

By the end of the chapter you will be able to:

- define critical appraisal and its role in evidence-based practice (EBP);
- discuss the steps required for critical appraisal in relation to different forms of evidence;
- understand the skills of critical appraisal;
- locate appropriate critical appraisal tools.

INTRODUCTION

Research is defined as 'The systematic investigation into and study of materials and sources in order to establish facts and reach new conclusions' (*Oxford English Dictionary*, 2018). Critical appraisal essentially means the assessment of the quality of a piece of research, and it is a key component of EBP. As such, it is a core skill for those engaged in reviewing or implementing new evidence. Much of what is written in this area relates to critical appraisal of published research literature. However, other types of evidence are fast emerging. It is essential that healthcare professionals critically appraise all evidence before integrating it into practice. Indeed, the requirement for engaging in research critique is becoming ever more apparent. In the UK, for example, the Nursing and Midwifery Council (NMC), the professional body that publishes, reviews and maintains standards for nursing and mid-wifery education and practice at both pre- and post-registration levels, published new standards for proficiency for nurses in May 2018. The standards clearly state how nurses must 'demonstrate an understanding of research methods, ethics and governance in order to critically analyse, safely use, share and apply research findings to promote and inform best nursing practice' and 'demonstrate the knowledge, skills and ability to think critically when applying evidence and drawing on experience to make evidence informed decisions in all situations' (NMC, 2018b). In this chapter, examples of tools that can help with this process are identified and the skills needed outlined.

WHAT IS CRITICAL APPRAISAL?

Critical means 'the objective analysis and evaluation of an issue in order to form a judgement' and appraisal is 'the act of assessing the worth, value or quality of a thing' (*Oxford English Dictionary*, 2018). Therefore, critical appraisal can be said to be a careful evaluation of the worth, value or quality of evidence. It is not only about identifying weaknesses in a piece of evidence but also about noting the strengths – critical appraisal should be an objective consideration of the merits and limitations of the evidence.

The end result of critical appraisal should be a balanced consideration of a study's validity and significance for practice; this will help with making decisions about how best to incorporate appropriate findings into practice.

CRITICAL APPRAISAL OF RESEARCH LITERATURE

Parkes et al. (2001: 1) defined critical appraisal as 'the process of assessing and interpreting evidence by systematically considering its validity, results and relevance to an individual's work'. They suggest that a basic understanding of research methods is essential when undertaking critical appraisal. It is, therefore, important that healthcare professionals develop a sound knowledge of the research process and its various components.

One of the problems with published work is people assume that because something is in print it must be high-quality evidence, but this may not always be the case. Although most research papers are subject to a rigorous peer review process – where experts have scrutinised the work and commented on its appropriateness for publication – not all published work is necessarily always of a high standard. Even when research is of high quality, most studies will still have some methodological weaknesses, as Nieswiadomy and Bailey (2017) identified; there is no such thing as a perfect research study, all have flaws or limitations of some sort. If research findings are to be used in practice it is vital those implementing them are aware of these limitations and consider their implications.

Polit and Beck (2018) have noted the frequent 'grey areas' in relation to some aspects of research, with experts having different opinions as to what they believe to be appropriate when conducting a study. As research methodologies develop and studies progress, researchers have to weigh up the differing opinions and issues relating to their area of interest and then make decisions about how to proceed with the research. This then has an impact on the overall research outcomes.

There are often compromises to be made in terms of what is considered ideal and what is practicable in the given situation. These compromises are often related to issues such as sample size, the methods used to collect and analyse data and/or the interpretation of findings. When critically appraising work these decisions can be evaluated by asking questions such as, 'Would another approach have been better?', 'Does the form of analysis have implications for the findings?' or 'Was the sample size sufficient to justify their conclusions?'. Decisions can then be made about the quality of the study as a whole and its relevance to clinical practice.

Issues related to the **validity**, **reliability**, **trustworthiness** and **relevance** of research studies are of prime importance to critical appraisal (Polit and Beck, 2018) and all of these concepts will be considered in more depth in later chapters. Briefly, however, validity relates to whether or not the claims made in a study are accurate; so, for instance, if the paper suggests its findings are generalisable, there is a need to consider if the methodology used supports such a claim. Reliability is concerned with identifying if the results are dependable and replicable and involves asking the question, 'If the research was repeated would the same results be found?' The concept of trustworthiness relates to whether data can be considered objective and credible. Establishing trustworthiness, particularly in qualitative research, has attracted much attention in recent years. Lincoln and Guba (1985) introduced trustworthiness criteria of credibility, transferability, dependability and confirmability (described in more depth in Chapter 8) to parallel the conventional quantitative assessment criteria of validity and reliability (discussed in more depth in Chapter 7). (See Nowell et al. (2017) for a useful example of how researchers have applied the Lincoln and Guba criteria to test the trustworthiness of their own qualitative research.) Finally, relevance is seen as a consideration as to whether the findings can be applied to the practice setting. Although these concepts are relevant to all forms of research, different criteria are often needed to make these judgements in relation to different research paradigms.

However, critical appraisal is based on the idea of **rigour**, which involves a judgement as to whether the research is of a high quality and whether measures were in place to ensure that the research was conducted in an appropriate way, consistent with the underpinning principles associated with the research paradigm.

Published research papers do tend to have a specific form, being organised into particular sections. Each of these sections is critically examined and certain aspects of each section are considered. The format of papers may vary slightly from journal to journal or appear in a different order when certain research approaches are used. Generally, the content remains the same, with all the aspects appearing in some form. There are, however, sometimes concerns about the quality of the reporting of research studies in journals. The EQUATOR (Enhancing the Quality and Transparency of Health Research) network has been set up to facilitate the development of reporting guidelines, which it is hoped will

Identify a topic of interest related to your recent clinical experience. Find two research articles related to the topic – one using a qualitative and one using a quantitative approach. Compare the articles' sections, identifying the similarities and the differences.

Visit the EQUATOR website at www.equator-network.org/home/ and identify if there are guidelines related to the methods from the chosen articles. If so, consider whether the articles meet the criteria identified.

Activity 6.1

improve transparency of studies and the accuracy of reporting. These have been created mainly for the use of authors, journal editors and peer reviewers and most researchers now use these approaches in designing and writing up their research studies. These guidelines can also aid the critical appraisal process.

A framework to critique research is offered by Polit and Beck (2018), which identifies the broad areas that should be considered in critical appraisal and are relevant to all forms of research (see Table 6.1). Parahoo (2014) suggests that the over-arching issues of sources of bias and omissions/exaggeration also need to be considered.

Bias is a distortion of the results and/or conclusions and can be introduced in a number of ways – from the participants, the researcher(s), methods of data collection, the environment and the phenomena under study. These will be considered in more depth in relation to qualitative and quantitative approaches in the following chapters.

Table 6.1 Elements for critique

Dimension	Issues to be considered
Substantive/ theoretical	Is this an important area to study?
	Does it have relevance to practice?
	Does it take knowledge in this area forward?
	Does the research approach fit with the question to be answered?
Methodological	Are the research design, sampling method, data collection tool and forms of analysis rigorous and appropriate to the research question/hypothesis?
Practical	Is the scope of the proposed research too broad?
	Have practical issues related to the actual 'doing' of the research been given consideration?
Ethical	Has the researcher identified the ethical issues associated with the research?
	Has ethical approval been sought and given?
Interpretive	Is the researcher's interpretation of the findings credible in light of the data?
	Does the researcher's interpretation appear logical when compared with your own understanding of the area and other research on the topic?
Presentation/ style	Is there enough information?
	Is it presented in a clear and concise way?
	Are the themes and arguments developed in a logical and reasoned way?

Exaggeration can result from authors over-emphasising the relevance of their results. For example, if people were asked whether they preferred jam or marmalade on their toast and 46 per cent said jam, you could say almost half of the people preferred jam, or fewer than half preferred jam; each statement implies something different in relation to the same result. Omissions generally fall into two categories – intentional and unintentional. The former is serious if there is an intention to deceive the reader by deliberately leaving out information that may identify flaws in the work. The latter are the most common and often a result of researchers being so familiar with their work that they forget that others may not have the same level of understanding. This often results in aspects of the study not being clearly explained or described. Also, in writing for publication, researchers will commonly experience problems in terms of the article length. Journals allow authors a fixed number of words, which may result in certain aspects being left out or minimal description being included.

Examine the two papers you chose for the preceding activity and identify any potential examples of exaggeration and/or omission in the papers. Consider the implications this might have in relation to the applicability of the studies to practice.

Activity 6.2

It is important to identify a study's methodology (though the details are normally – or should usually be – explicitly stated by the authors) before you begin to critically appraise an article so that you can find an appropriate appraisal tool to help with the process. Once the methods have been established, the next step involves identifying the most appropriate checklist to assist with the process. There are a large number of tools available both in books and online which have been designed specifically to help (non-expert) researchers and clinicians appraise the quality of evidence emerging from a range of different study types. Indeed, an increasing number of organisations are publishing resources to support the critical appraisal process. It is crucial to choose the correct tool as each gives standard items on a checklist which have been selected in order to assess the relative strengths and weaknesses of a particular study design. A number of tools are available to download free of charge and Table 6.2 details those available from two key organisations, the Critical Appraisal Skills Programme (CASP) and the Joanna Briggs Institute (JBI). All tools have the common aim of aiding in the process of assessing the quality of published literature.

Additionally, the Centre for Evidence-Based Medicine has published a range of tools and other resources for the critical appraisal of different types of medical evidence. Example appraisal sheets are provided together with examples of how to apply them (see www.cebm.net/2014/06/critical-appraisal/). Specifically for Mixed Methods Studies, McGill University has published an appraisal tool, which can be used with permission (see http://mixedmethodsappraisaltoolpublic.pbworks. com/w/file/fetch/84371689/MMAT%202011%20criteria%20and%20tutorial%20 2011-06-29updated2014.08.21.pdf).

Table 6.2   Example of critical appraisal tools

Published by the Critical Appraisal Skills Programme (CASP) (available at: www.casp-uk.net/).	Published by The Joanna Briggs Institute (JBI) (available at: http://joannabriggs.org/research/critical-appraisal-tools.html)
CASP tools are currently available for the critical appraisal of:	JBI tools are currently available for the critical appraisal of:
• Systematic reviews • Qualitative studies • Randomised controlled trials • Case control studies • Cohort studies • Clinical prediction rules • Diagnostic test studies • Economic evaluations	• Systematic reviews • Qualitative studies • Randomised controlled trials • Case control studies • Cohort studies • Case reports • Case series • Diagnostic test accuracy studies • Economic evaluations • Prevalence studies • Quasi-experimental studies (non-randomised experimental studies) • Text and opinion • Analytical cross-sectional studies

Although qualitative and quantitative approaches are fundamentally different they do have some common areas for consideration and these are discussed below. Appendix 4 provides a tool containing general criteria to consider when critiquing an article in this way.

Activity 6.3

Identify the methodological approach used in each of your chosen research studies. Using any of the resources above, find an appropriate appraisal tool for each of the studies.

Research design

The research design is the overall plan for the research, and should be coherent and appropriate to answer the research question under investigation. One particular area for consideration is that of patient and/or public involvement. Just as there is increasing emphasis on the need to ensure the user's voice is heard in the organisation and delivery of care, so too has user involvement become central to the research process, not simply as participants but rather as part of the whole process. Indeed, in the UK, the Health Research Authority (HRA) has set out its commitment that 'patients, service users and the public are given, and take, the opportunity to participate in health and social care research and to get involved in its design, management, conduct and dissemination, and are confident about doing so' (HRA, 2018: 4). Furthermore, a central resource has been funded by the National Institute for Health Research to support public involvement in research (available at: www.invo.org.uk).

INVOLVE was established in 1996 and is part of, and funded by, the National Institute for Health Research, to support active public involvement in NHS, public health and social care research. It is one of the few government-funded programmes of its kind in the world.

Take some time to explore its website (www.invo.org.uk/) to gain a fuller understanding into the ways in which members of the public can bring expertise, insight and experience to the research process.

Activity 6.4

Literature review

In most published studies, a review of contextual literature is usually present. It should be up to date, and relevant to the research question/hypothesis and proposed objective/aims. Parahoo (2014) suggests four criteria by which to judge a literature review:

1. Whether it provides a rationale for the study. The review should identify why it is important the study is undertaken, the benefits and possible outcomes.
2. Whether it puts the current study into context. It should consider what is already known about the concepts under consideration and provide a balanced view of the various debates around the chosen focus.
3. Whether it provides a review of research relevant to the topic. Research previously conducted should be considered and conclusions drawn, and implications for the proposed study identified.
4. Whether it provides a conceptual/theoretical framework for the research. As you will see below, not all research identifies a theoretical and conceptual framework; however, a literature review should provide an overview of the different frameworks available.

Theoretical/conceptual framework

The purpose of research is to generate new knowledge, which involves the testing, adjusting and developing of theories. Therefore, there is a need to identify what theory underpins or guides the research process. The terms theoretical framework and conceptual framework are often used interchangeably, although there are distinctions between them – the former usually refers to the use of one theory whereas the latter generally involves the combining of concepts from a range of theories. As Parahoo (2014) has suggested, in practice this distinction is not always recognised by researchers. In fact, this aspect is frequently missing or only mentioned in passing in research reports. It may, however, remain implicit within the literature review, the operational definitions or the discussion of the findings in relation to other literature.

Ethical issues

All health service research undertaken in UK care organisations has required formal ethical approval since the Research Governance Framework became law in 2004. Since then, the Health Research Authority (HRA) and the Devolved UK Administrations developed a new UK Policy Framework for Health and Social Care Research which sets out the high-level principles of good practice in the management and conduct of health and social care research in the UK, as well as the responsibilities that underpin high-quality ethical research (HRA, 2018). The regulations governing other countries may vary but the underlying principles are generally the same, reflecting the World Medical Association's (2004) *Declaration of Helsinki* concerning the ethical principles health professionals should consider (see www.wma.net/policies-post/wma-declaration-of-helsinki-ethical-principles-for-medical-research-involving-human-subjects/). Although not legally binding the declaration has been a major influence on the development of legislation relating to research ethics across the world.

Population

The population is the particular group of people that a researcher is interested in and needs to be specifically described. It could be people with a learning disability who have a particular challenging behaviour or children between the ages of 10 and 16 years who have appendicitis. It refers to the entire group; however, data are not usually collected from the entire population, rather a sample is selected (see below).

Sampling

This term describes the process used to identify the segment of the population invited to take part in the study. People who form the sample within quantitative research are generally termed **subjects** or **sampling units**. Generally, the word **participant** is used in relation to those who take part in qualitative research. This reflects the basic philosophy that individuals take an active role in the research process, rather than being passive subjects. Different ways of identifying the sample are used in qualitative and quantitative research and are discussed in more detail in Chapters 7 and 8.

Pilot study

Often before the full research study is carried out, a small 'pilot' study will be conducted to test out the design and forms of data collection. This allows for any adjustments to be made to the main study prior to implementation. For example, the questions in a questionnaire may be changed if they are found to be unclear or ambiguous when tested on a small group first.

Data collection, analysis and results

These areas relate to the type of information that has been collected, and how it was gathered, processed, analysed and reported. This will be discussed in more depth in the following chapters.

Discussion

Polit and Beck (2018) have argued that the discussion should address the main findings of the study and what they mean, consider evidence to support the validity of the findings and examine what limitations may impact on this validity. There is also a need to consider the findings in light of what is already known about the topic under investigation.

Applicability to practice

Finally, applicability relates to whether research findings can be implemented in a particular practice setting. To judge applicability sufficient information must be present within the evidence to identify whether the population sampled in the study is comparable with the population identified in the clinical literature review question. Information related to age, cultural beliefs and values, ethnicity and lifestyle is essential if a judgement is to be made. As with any form of research, while there may be evidence that a particular treatment is effective, there is still a need to consider it in light of specific patient preferences. Interestingly, the new NMC standards for nurse education in the UK specifically noted the need for nurses to understand the requirement to base all decisions regarding care and interventions on people's needs and preferences, recognising and addressing any personal and external factors that may unduly influence their decisions (NMC, 2018b).

CRITIQUING CLINICAL GUIDELINES

Clinical guidelines are documents which aim to guide decisions and criteria regarding diagnosis, management and treatment in specific areas of healthcare and are now readily available on a wide range of topics. In the UK, clinical practice guidelines are published primarily by the National Institute for Health and Care Excellence (NICE; www.nice.org.uk/). They are based on the best available evidence and include recommendations by experts, people using services, carers and the public. NICE has published a very useful document outlining the details of the transparency and inclusiveness of the process for the development of UK clinical guidelines (NICE, 2009). Clinical guidelines have become an important aspect of clinical governance as they promote clinical and cost effectiveness and provide a bridge between research and practice.

Sanderlin and Abdul Rahhim (2007) have offered guidance for critiquing clinical practice guidelines, suggesting that while these are important tools in promoting EBP there are various issues to be considered before implementing them. These relate to:

- strength of evidence;
- objective approach to development of guidelines;

- homogeneity of studies – based on studies that have similar designs and complementary results;
- whether study subjects are significantly similar to the relevant patient group;
- whether the guidelines are based on evidence that has been appropriately appraised.

While clinical guidelines are a useful aid to increasing the use of research in the delivery and management of care, they are not without problems and this has been recognised for some time. Bugers et al. (2002), for example, reviewed 15 clinical guidelines from 13 countries on type 2 diabetes. Although there was overall general agreement in terms of management of the disease, some differences in terms of treatment were identified. They found that the guidelines' recommendations shared little common evidence, with only 1 per cent of evidence appearing in six or more of the guidelines. This lack of common ground highlights the need to give careful consideration to guidelines before using them in practice.

In an effort to address these issues, processes for guideline development are being generated to ensure that they are produced in a rigorous and appropriate manner.

Many organisations now request that in compiling clinical guidelines developers use the Grades of Recommendation, Assessment, Development and Evaluation (GRADE) process (see www.gradeworkinggroup.org/). This approach provides guidance on how to rate the quality of evidence and strength of recommendations. It provides a 'systematic and transparent framework' for developing guidelines (Guyatt et al., 2011: 380). Guidelines produced using the GRADE approach indicate whether recommendations are based on strong or weak evidence and, therefore, give an indication of the merits of the evidence used. It may be helpful when critically appraising guidelines to identify whether or not the GRADE approach has been used.

The Appraisal of Guidelines Research and Evaluation Collaboration, now the AGREE Research Trust (www.agreetrust.org/), provides a tool for appraising clinical guidelines. This international collaboration's aim is to improve the quality and effectiveness of guidelines by promoting a common approach to their development and assessment. The AGREE tool was updated and AGREE II launched in 2009, consisting of 23 criteria organised in six domains. The AGREE Research Trust proposes that the instrument can be used to assess all forms of guidelines (local, national, international) with the exception of quality guidance related to healthcare organisation issues, and provides a user's manual to help people with the process of appraisal.

Activity 6.5

Identify a set of guidelines you recently used in practice. Consider these against the AGREE II criteria at www.agreetrust.org. Consider whether or not the guidelines meet the AGREE II criteria.

SKILLS OF CRITICAL APPRAISAL

It is important to remember that the skills of critical appraisal are developed over time, and get easier with practice. Critically appraising something takes time; it shouldn't be a rushed activity, as it requires careful study, checking the information provided, and possibly consulting other people and sources of information.

The first thing to consider is whether the evidence is from a credible source. If it comes from a journal there are generally some checks already in place – most journals will identify whether or not they subject submissions to peer review. As identified in Chapter 5 there are already some sources of pre-appraised evidence available.

Internet sources do not always have such checks in place; for example, self-publishing sites such as Wikis may have little or no control over the information placed on the web page or its trustworthiness. Decisions will need to be taken as to whether the site is credible – checking an organisation's credentials or asking others what they know about certain sites are useful activities. Box 6.1 gives some examples of what to look for when making a judgement as to a website's credibility. This may save unnecessary work if the source is later found not to be reputable.

Box 6.1   Judging the credibility/reliability of a website

Check:

- the URL – if it contains a tilde (~) this means it's been created by an individual and therefore is less likely to be credible;
- the domain name, e.g.

  - com = commercial – may be biased
  - co.uk = commercial – may be biased
  - ac.uk = university – likely to be reliable
  - edu = education – likely to be reliable
  - gov = government – likely to be reliable;

- the site's publication/update date – the more recent the more likely it is to be accurate;
- the purpose of the site – is it trying to sell something? If so, it may be biased (it is important to be able to make a judgement about whether the quality of the evidence is sufficiently robust to inform clinical decision making). There are many excellent websites where the content is targeted at patients or the general population. While these serve a valuable purpose in terms of information dissemination, using this information to inform decision making directly, without seeking out the *original* source of evidence, is not recommended.

(Continued)

(Continued)

- the contact details – these should be present and authenticity can be checked by 'googling' them for further details;
- whether the site is affiliated to an identified group (university, government, healthcare agency)? If so, it is likely to be more credible;
- the stated objective of the site – this may give an indication of the site's purpose and relevance;
- the information on the website – is it verified by other sources?
- the quality of writing – a large number of spelling/grammatical errors probably means it is less reliable;
- the quality of the citations it contains, or evidence it presents.

Greenhalgh (2014) has suggested beginning the actual appraisal process by 'getting your bearings' and asking three broad questions:

1. What clinical question is being answered?
2. What type of study is it?
3. Is the design appropriate to the area of research?

By asking these questions decisions can be taken as to whether or not to continue with the appraisal of a particular piece of evidence. If the evidence does not address a question of interest, there is no point in continuing. Identifying the type of study helps with locating an appropriate tool for critique of the work. The appropriateness of the approach is essential in answering clinical questions. If the area of interest is the effectiveness of an intervention but the approach used is one more suitable to considering the feasibility of using a particular intervention then, once again, there is no point in appraising the study. If the study meets all three of these criteria, then the next step is to undertake a full appraisal.

A similar approach known as 'Rapid Critical Appraisal' is put forward by Fineout-Overholt et al. (2010a). Here it is suggested that the following key areas are considered:

1. Type of study and place within a hierarchy of evidence.
2. How well it was conducted.
3. Applicability to practice.

In this approach a particular level of evidence is being examined; that is, RCTs. Therefore, the placing of the evidence within a hierarchy is essential. In steps 2 and 3 Fineout-Overholt et al. (2010b) advocated a consideration of the results and their validity and their relevance to the appraiser's own area of practice. Only if a paper meets the criteria related to appropriate levels of evidence, valid results and apparent applicability to practice is it taken forward for full critical appraisal.

The Royal College of Nursing (a professional body supporting nurses across the UK) has collated a list of resources aimed at supporting health professionals to read research papers through a critical lens.

Take some time to explore the link below and familiarise yourself with key tips pertaining to each of the difference types of research study.

www.bmj.com/about-bmj/resources-readers/publications/how-read-paper

Activity 6.6

To critically appraise evidence a step-by-step approach, as outlined below, will need to be followed, but as confidence and skills grow practitioners also tend to develop their own systems.

1. Identify a suitable checklist to use to critically appraise the evidence.
2. Find somewhere quiet, where you are unlikely to be interrupted.
3. Read through the paper once, so you have a grasp of the content.
4. Read through it again in more depth, evaluating each part of the paper.
5. Make notes or highlight important bits of the paper as you go along.
6. Have a research book to hand so you can check out information or fill in any gaps in your knowledge as you read.
7. Complete the appraisal and discuss your findings with others.

There are resources available to help develop skills in this area such as Critical Appraisal Topics (CATs). These are summaries of evidence relating to a clinical question generated in response to a specific clinical problem (Foster et al., 2001). Originally a paper-based exercise generated by McMaster University in Canada to encourage medical students to develop critical appraisal skills, CATs created by various individuals are available online as a possible resource and learning tool for other health professionals. An electronic tool known as a CAT-maker created by the NHS Research and Development Centre for Evidence-based Medicine at Oxford is also freely available to help with the generation of CATs. Although this has been developed for the medical profession, the process can also be of use to others in the healthcare setting as it can provide a summary of the evidence and ends with a judgement as to its appropriateness to address the question asked.

Visit the Centre for Evidence-based Medicine CAT-maker website at www.cebm.net/. Download the tool and consider whether this would be a useful tool in conducting critical appraisals.

Activity 6.7

CATs are a useful learning tool as they:

- provide an example of critical appraisal in relation to a live issue using accessible evidence sources;
- provide a concise step–by–step method for recording the process of critical appraisal which can then be shared with others;
- help in the development of critical appraisal skills;
- enable a structured and informed approach to clinical decision making.

However, CATs are not without their disadvantages. They have a limited life span unless they are regularly updated and may contain errors due to a lack of individual knowledge or particular forms of interpretation.

It is useful to have an overview of the details of the literature, particularly if there are a number of studies which may not be fully appropriate to a specific area of interest. The easiest way to do this is to generate a summary table of the various studies' details (see Appendix 5 for an example). This will be useful when later making decisions about integrating evidence into practice.

In developing the skills associated with critical appraisal it is important to remember that to become proficient takes time and that no one is expected to know everything or get it completely right the first time. It is important to know how to find the information needed to conduct the appraisal and to discuss findings with others and ask for their opinions.

Activity 6.8

Choose one of the papers identified earlier. Using the appropriate critical appraisal tool undertake a critical appraisal of the paper identifying the aspects/questions you are able to fully critique and those where you need to develop further skills and knowledge. Develop an action plan outlining how you will develop the knowledge and skills you require to complete the task appropriately.

Summary

- Critical appraisal is associated with published research literature, but there is a need to appraise all forms of evidence.
- Critical appraisal should be an objective consideration of the merits and limitations of the evidence.
- Not all published work is of an appropriate standard or applicable to the practice setting, therefore critical appraisal is a key aspect of EBP.
- Skills of critical appraisal take time to develop and practice is essential.

FURTHER READING

Greenhalgh, T. (2014) *How to Read a Paper: The Basics of Evidence-Based Medicine* (5th edn). Oxford: John Wiley & Sons/BMJ Books.

Health Research Authority (HRA) (2018) *UK Policy Framework for Health and Social Care Research*. Health Research Authority.

Parahoo, K. (2014) *Nursing Research: Principles, Process and Issues* (3rd edn). Basingstoke: Palgrave Macmillan. This book provides an excellent introduction to the research process.

USEFUL WEBLINKS

Critical Appraisal Skills Programme: provides a range of resources to help with developing the skills associated with EBP. It also provides a range of critical appraisal tools. www.casp-uk.net

The Health Research Authority (HRA) is a body of the Department of Health in the UK, set up to protect and promote the interests of patients and the public in health and social care research. It has published or made available a number of key resources about good research practice including the ADASS/SSRG resource pack for social care, the ESRC Framework for Research Ethics, the principles of ICH GCP, the previous Research Governance Frameworks, the RESPECT Code of Practice, the UUK Concordat to support research integrity and the WMA Declaration of Helsinki. See: www.hra.nhs.uk/planning-and-improving-research/policies-standards-legislation/uk-policy-framework-health-social-care-research

The Joanna Briggs Institute (JBI) is an international not-for-profit, research and development centre within the Faculty of Health and Medical Sciences at the University of Adelaide, South Australia, which provides a wide range of resources to support researchers including a range of tools to aid critical appraisal. See: http://joannabriggs.org/research/critical-appraisal-tools.html

The National Institute for Health and Care Excellence: provides national guidance on preventing and treating illness and promoting health. www.nice.org.uk. Specifically in relation to the development of Clinical Guidelines, see: www.nice.org.uk/about/what-we-do/our-programmes/nice-guidance/nice-guidelines/how-we-develop-nice-guidelines

The Royal College of Nursing in the UK provides useful links to resources to aid and inform critical appraisal of evidence. www.rcn.org.uk/library/subject-guides. Specifically: www.rcn.org.uk/library/subject-guides/critical-appraisal and www.rcn.org.uk/library/subject-guides/doing-your-dissertation

7

Critical Appraisal and Quantitative Research

Janet Barker, Ros Kane and David Nelson

Learning Outcomes

By the end of the chapter you will be able to:

- provide an overview of quantitative research approaches;
- identify the key areas for consideration when critically appraising quantitative literature;
- discuss different sampling strategies and methods of analysis used in quantitative research;
- debate issues of reliability and validity.

INTRODUCTION

Quantitative research is primarily concerned with examining how different variables interact and impact on each other. Mantzoukas (2008) found that 51 per cent of research studies published in the top 10 generic nursing journals (such as the *Journal of Advanced Nursing* and the *Journal of Clinical Nursing*) were quantitative in nature. Thus, it is crucial that nurses and other healthcare professionals have a solid understanding of the principles of quantitative research and how to interpret findings from a range of different types of quantitative study.

This chapter briefly outlines some methods used in quantitative research and discusses the issues to be considered when critically appraising quantitative literature. However, it is not intended to provide a full overview of quantitative research, and for a more in-depth exploration you will need to consider some of the recommended reading at the end of the chapter.

WHAT IS QUANTITATIVE RESEARCH?

As identified in Chapter 2, quantitative research has its roots in positivism and in using a deductive approach, starting with a theoretical framework or conceptual model, which predicts how things (**variables**) behave in the world. Specific predictions (hypotheses) are then deduced from the theory and tested (Polit and Beck, 2018). The aim of quantitative research is, therefore, to explore the relationships between variables and to test hypotheses. It uses objective, rigorous and systematic approaches. A researcher will identify the variables of interest, clearly define what these are and then collect data usually in a numerical form.

A variable, simply put, is something that varies from one person/situation to another. So weight, temperature, pain and personality traits are all variables. Quantitative research seeks to understand why these variations occur. For example, high blood pressure is a variable as not everyone experiences it. If a variable is extremely varied within a particular group it is said to be heterogeneous and where there is limited variability it is described as being homogeneous. Table 7.1 outlines some different types of variables.

Table 7.1   Types of variable

Type	Description
Dependent	The focus of the research (the study is usually conducted to understand the influences on the dependent variable) The factor/characteristic or behaviour that the researcher is attempting to understand, describe or affect
Independent	The factor/characteristic or behaviour that is considered to have an influence on the dependent variable
Confounding	A variable that correlates with both the dependent and independent variable. A significant association between the dependent and independent variable may be occurring simply because of the two variables being associated with the confounding variable (also known as a confounding factor or confounder)

Usually, in a quantitative study, the focus is on examining the relationship between independent and dependent variables. For example, you could consider whether age (independent variable) has any implications for the onset of high blood pressure (dependent variable). Whether a variable is identified as dependent or independent depends on the focus of the study. In the above example high blood pressure is the dependent variable, and age is the independent variable. A further study could be conducted to investigate whether there is an association between high blood pressure and other health outcomes such as incidence of coronary artery disease. In this case, high blood pressure would be the independent variable and occurrence of coronary artery disease the dependent variable.

Polit and Beck (2018) suggest quantitative research generally considers specific questions about the relationships, such as:

- the relationship between variables – e.g. is body weight related to the onset of type 2 diabetes?
- the direction of a relationship between variables – e.g. is someone who is overweight more or less likely to develop type 2 diabetes?
- the strength of the relationship between variables – e.g. how likely is it that someone who is overweight will develop type 2 diabetes?
- the cause and effect relationship between the variables – e.g. does being overweight cause the development of type 2 diabetes?

A key element of quantitative research is to determine whether any noted association between two variables is actually a causative association or one that has simply occurred by chance.

Usually a hypothesis is generated providing a simple statement of the variables to be considered and the relationship between them. For example, I could hypothesise that providing play activities (independent variable) for children prior to surgery will reduce their anxiety (dependent variable). A study could then be designed and conducted to test this hypothesis.

Activity 7.1

Consider an issue that is causing concern in your area of practice. Identify the variables that might be considered in a study and generate a hypothesis as to the relationship between them.

Sample size is an important consideration in quantitative studies. Put simply, the larger the sample, the more power a study has to detect associations which are statistically significant. For more in-depth reading about sample size calculations please refer to the recommended reading at the end of the chapter. Usually a large number of people are recruited into quantitative research studies, and statistical tests are used to analyse the data and enable these to be presented in a succinct form. Statistics also help in making judgements regarding the level of statistical significance of research findings.

Analysis is an attempt to measure the concepts and variables under consideration as accurately and objectively as possible. Objectivity is seen as a central tenet of quantitative research, with the researcher viewed as 'standing outside' the research process. The intention here is to ensure that neither the researcher nor the subjects introduce any form of bias into the research process. Bias is where the results of a study are distorted for some reason (this, along with ways to reduce bias, will be considered in more detail later in the chapter). To reduce bias a process known as blinding is often used. Here information relating to the research process is concealed from those on whom the research is conducted and/or those involved in delivering the intervention being studied. For example, if the effectiveness of a particular drug is being tested, an experimental group of subjects receive the drug and a control group receive a placebo. The subjects and/or those administering the drug may not be made aware of who is receiving it and who is receiving the placebo. If information is withheld from only one of the groups involved – the subjects or those administering the drug – it is called a single-blind study. If information is withheld from both groups it would be known as a double-blind study.

TYPES OF QUANTITATIVE RESEARCH

Generally, two types of research design are present within quantitative research: experimental and non-experimental.

Experimental approaches, such as randomised control trials (RCTs), actively introduce a treatment or intervention in an attempt to study causal relationships. The aim is to identify whether a particular intervention has an impact on the dependent variable. To be a true experimental design the following three conditions must be met:

1. An intervention is controlled by a researcher so some subjects receive the intervention and others do not.
2. At least two groups of subjects are involved – a control group and an experimental group.
3. Random selection and allocation of subjects to research groups will occur.

If these three conditions are not all met, the research is described as quasi-experimental. Quasi-experimental approaches are used to test the effectiveness of interventions and are often done when it is not possible to meet one of the three conditions above.

Concerns have been raised in relation to the quality of the reporting of experimental studies. It is suggested that frequently the information given is not sufficient to allow proper critical appraisal. To address these concerns, guidelines as to what should be included in reports of RCTs have been generated; these are known as the CONSORT (Consolidated Standards of Reporting Trials) statement (Schulz et al., 2010). Various 'extensions' to the CONSORT statement have been developed to give guidance on specific designs, data and interventions. Statements related to other forms of quantitative research are also being developed. These may be of help in identifying what should be included in quantitative research studies.

Visit the CONSORT website at www.consort-statement.org and use the CONSORT statement to identify the aspects that are considered to be central to the designing and writing up of randomised control trials (RCTs).

Activity 7.2

Non-experimental quantitative research is used to describe and/or identify associations between variables and would generally be used to address Polit and Beck's (2018) first three questions (see above). However, it is not possible to definitively establish cause and effect relationships. Instead, the intention is to explore potential associations – possibly with a view to establishing firm causative relationships in future research. Key examples of non-experimental study designs are outlined below.

Cross-sectional studies collect data at a single point in time (for example, by doing a survey of a population). They may also be used to make comparisons between different groups within that population. For example, if you wanted to measure whether the length of time someone was in residential care impacts on their level of satisfaction, you might collect data at the same point from current residents, ask how long they had been in residential care and compare levels of satisfaction between those who had lived in the setting for three months, six months, nine months and twelve months.

Longitudinal studies (also known as cohort studies) collect data at various points over an extended period of time from an identified individual/group of people. For example, if you were interested in the impact of socioeconomic factors on the health outcomes of children from birth to the age of six you would collect data from the same group of children from birth to the age of six years at defined intervals (perhaps at six-month intervals).

Retrospective studies collect data after an event and look back or ask questions relating to historical situations. For example, patients' notes may be examined for information in relation to a specific treatment and recovery. It is possible to make comparisons between two different groups (case control studies), such as those who developed a particular disease and those who remained free from disease.

Prospective studies collect data in relation to a specific independent variable and the dependent variable is measured at a later date. In this approach it would be possible, for example, to consider if coping behaviours in relation to stress have an impact on incidence of myocardial infarctions by measuring stress-coping behaviours in a population and then identifying the number of people who had a myocardial infarction in 10 years' time.

It is important to differentiate between **descriptive** and **correlation studies**. Descriptive studies generally observe, describe and document areas of interest as they occur naturally. Correlation studies examine relationships between variables. Again, as identified in relation to RCTs, reporting guidelines have been created with regard to a number of these approaches and can be found at the EQUATOR network website (www.equator-network.org/).

CRITICAL APPRAISAL

As identified in Chapter 6, there are a number of tools available to help you critically appraise the different types of quantitative research. Therefore, it is important to use the correct checklist to help you focus on the most important aspects of the study. Appendix 6 gives a generic approach to particular areas to be addressed in this form of critique – those specific to quantitative research are highlighted, and an overview is given below. For discussion of the other general items see Chapter 6. Remember, when doing a critical appraisal it is helpful to have a good research book to hand so information can be clarified along the way.

> Find a quantitative research study relevant to your area of practice and an appropriate critical appraisal tool.
>
> **Activity 7.3**

Hypothesis/research question and research objectives/aims

Not all quantitative research has a hypothesis, particularly descriptive studies. However, there should always be a clearly stated research question. If a hypothesis is required this should be a simple statement identifying the relationship between at least two clearly stated variables and it should be testable. Different types of hypotheses include the following:

- Directional – suggests the nature and direction of the relationship between variables: positive (e.g. increased physical activity improves mental functioning); inverse/negative (e.g. people with learning disabilities display less challenging behaviour when involved in diversional activities); difference (e.g. people with high blood pressure are more likely to suffer from a coronary artery disease than those who do not have high blood pressure).
- Non-directional – this only suggests that a relationship might exist (e.g. children differ from adults in the levels of anxiety they experience on admission to hospital).
- Null hypothesis – where no relationship is suggested (e.g. there is no relationship between the use of cognitive behavioural therapy and an improvement of mood in people who are depressed).

The aims/objectives of the research should also be clearly identified and reflect the research question and/or hypothesis.

Operational definitions

It is expected that concepts used within the research will be defined. For example, if a study related to whether wound dressing X is more effective than wound dressing Y in the treatment of leg ulcers, there is a need to clearly define what is meant by wound dressings X and Y, leg ulcer, the procedures to be used when applying the dressing and the effects to be measured. While words such as 'leg ulcer' are in common usage, within the research context there is a need to identify precisely what type of leg ulcers are to be considered. Without this type of information the rigour and the generalisability of the findings can be called into question and the ability to identify if the research is relevant to a specific area of practice is compromised.

> **Activity 7.4**
>
> Read the article chosen in the previous activity. Identify the operational definitions and appraise whether these are sufficiently described to allow you to identify applicability to your own area of practice.

Data collection methods

The measurement tools selected to collect data must be appropriate to the research question/ hypothesis and the operational definitions and should also collect the type and level of data required. Data collection methods in quantitative research can take many forms – questionnaires, observational schedules, self-reporting schedules or bio-physiological measures. All of these approaches involve the measurement of variables through the assignment of numbers to the variable according to pre-agreed rules. For example, there are identified rules and methods for measuring weight, which allow you to observe what someone weighs. However, not all variables are easily measured and methods of measurement have to be agreed to allow measurement to be taken.

In considering measurement in quantitative research there is a need to understand:

- what is being measured;
- how it is being measured;
- why it is being measured in this way;
- what the rules are in relation to that measurement (Parahoo, 2014).

Without this information it is not possible to judge whether the data being collected are accurate.

There are two main criteria for assessing the research tools – reliability and validity, which are both discussed in more detail below. However, briefly, reliability of measurement tools relates to the accuracy with which a tool measures the variable, whether it is able to reproduce findings consistently and be free from error. Validity relates to whether the tool measures what it is meant to measure. Frequently, researchers use tools that have already been tested for reliability and validity. If a new tool is being used then there should be evidence that it has been pre-tested for its reliability/validity.

Data collection protocols are usually produced by quantitative researchers identifying procedures for collecting data. Clear instructions as to what conditions should be met and any specific instruction in relation to the sequencing of collecting and recording of information are expected to be present.

Sampling

Studies almost always involve samples rather than the whole population of interest. If findings are to be generalised to the population of interest, then the sample must be representative of the whole of that population. The sample size required for a particular study is often determined through the use of power calculations. Statistical power is the ability of a study to detect statistically significant results. The power of a test is affected by the sample size, and power calculations will identify the sample size needed to detect significant differences where they exist. A well-designed study will identify the use of power calculations in calculating sample sizes.

Quantitative research generally uses what is known as probability sampling. In this type of sample every unit within the population of interest has an equal chance of being selected. To ensure representativeness, random selection procedures are used. Appropriate randomisation is of central importance as it ensures that neither the researchers nor the subjects will be able to influence characteristics of the population under study. Four approaches to probability sampling are available – simple, stratified, systematic and cluster (see Table 7.2).

Table 7.2   Types of randomised sampling

Type	Description
Simple random sampling	A sampling frame is generated listing all the elements of the population
	A number is allocated to each one of the elements
	A table of random grouped numbers (computer generated) is used to select sample units for specified sample size
Stratified random sampling	Ensures subgroups (e.g. age, ethnicity) within a population are present in the sample in the same proportions
	Proportional stratified sampling = sample proportions are same as population
	Disproportional sampling = a large sample of a particular subgroup is needed to consider the relationship between variables in that group
	Weighting = adjustments made to statistical analysis to provide actual population values
	Simple random sampling used to select the subjects from each subgroup
Cluster random (multi-stage) sampling	Used in large-scale studies with a widespread geographical population
	Clusters of target population randomly selected
	Units within each cluster again randomly selected to be part of the sample
	Simple random sampling would be used at each stage

(Continued)

Table 7.2   (Continued)

Type	Description
Systematic random sampling	Sample units are selected at predetermined intervals, e.g. every 5th or 7th or 20th unit on sampling frame
	Interval used decided by dividing the available target population by the sample size required, e.g. 100 units for a sample of 20 = every 5th unit selected (100 · 20 = 5)
	Sample frame itself is randomised before using this form of sampling

It is important that clear and precise accounts of the inclusion and exclusion criteria are documented within the study in order that the exact characteristics of the population used for the collection of data are known. Inclusion criteria are characteristics that the prospective subjects must have if they are to be included in the study, while exclusion criteria are those characteristics that disqualify prospective subjects from inclusion in the study. Without this information, the generalisability of findings to other client groups will be called into question, therefore reducing your ability to make decisions as to the applicability of the research to your own area of practice.

Data analysis

Statistical analysis allows quantitative researchers to make sense of the mass of numbers generated in the collection of data. There are four levels of data within quantitative research – nominal, ordinal, interval and ratio (see Box 7.1). The level of data indicates the statistical test to be used. It is beyond the scope of this chapter to give a full account of all forms of data test and analysis. However, some books are recommended at the end of this chapter.

Zellner et al. (2007) having reviewed over 400 research articles in various nursing journals found that 80 per cent of these used the same 10 statistical approaches (see Box 7.2 for a description of these 10 approaches). Further books on study design and statistical techniques are recommended at the end of this chapter.

Box 7.1   Levels of measurement of variables

- *Nominal* Simply categorises groups (e.g. male or female) and assigns a code number to the identifying traits, for example, Male = 1, Female = 2. Allows the identification of the frequency of a trait within a category – for example, identifying that 60 per cent of a sample were female.
- *Ordinal* Codes information according to an order in relation to specified criteria. Likert scales produce ordinal data (e.g. strongly agree, agree, neither agree nor disagree, disagree, strongly disagree).
- *Interval* Rank ordering of characteristics, in which the distance between any two numbers on the scale is known (e.g. temperature scale).
- *Ratio* Ordering of a trait, the intervals between each rank and the absolute magnitude of the trait (e.g. height or weight).

Box 7.2   Description of statistical tests most commonly used in nursing and health research

Descriptive statistics

- *Mean* – the average sum of a set of values. If the ages of six people were identified as 26, 29, 30, 38, 40 and 41, the mean age would be 34: (26 + 29 + 30 + 38 + 40 + 41 = 204 · 6 = 34).
- *Frequency distribution* – the arrangement of data in ascending order (lowest to highest value), identifying the number of times a particular value or score occurs. If the stress levels of 50 people prior to surgery were measured and given a numerical score (ranging from 1 to 10) it might result in the following frequency distribution:

  o   Frequency 2 3 5 8 11 7 6 4 3 1 (n 50)
  o   Score 1 2 3 4 5 6 7 8 9 10

- *Standard deviation* – the average deviation of the values from the mean.
- *Range* – the distance between highest and lowest values and gives a picture of the dispersion of data (the range between 15 per cent and 85 per cent = 70).
- *Percentages, percentiles and quartiles* – the frequency at which something occurs is reported in percentages, e.g. 60 per cent of people prefer butter to margarine; a percentile is the point below which a specific percentage of values lies (a score at a 60th percentile means 60 per cent of scores are below that); quartiles divide distribution scores into four equal parts.

Inferential statistics

- *t-test* – examines the difference between the means of two sets of values.
- *Analysis of variant* (ANOVA) – examines the difference between several means.
- *Correlation* – identifies an association between variables where a variation in one is related to a variation in another.
- *Cronbach's alpha* – a reliability index used to measure internal consistency of a multi-itemed measurement tool such as an anxiety scale or an assessment tool.
- *Chi-squared* – compares data collected in the form of frequencies or percentages.

Briefly, statistics are identified as being either descriptive or inferential. Descriptive statistics, as the term suggests, 'describe' and summarise the data, often in the form of averages and percentages. Within the EBP movement one of the most useful forms of descriptive statistics in decision making are effect/risk measures. These measures are used to calculate the 'clinical meaningfulness' of findings and are frequently seen in systematic reviews. However, these are also being increasingly included in research reports and it may be useful for you to explore these in more depth.

Inferential statistics allow researchers to make 'inferences' (draw conclusions) about the specific relationships between variables. The type of test used usually depends on:

- the sampling method;
- the level of data required (e.g. nominal);
- the distribution of variables to be measured.

Parametric tests are usually adopted where the sample is randomised, where there is a normal distribution of variables. These types of test are generally seen to be more powerful that non-parametric tests. Non-parametric tests do not consider a particular form of distribution to be present, and can be used with nominal and also ordinal data and on small samples.

Statistical tests that identify significance – whether an observed result is the product of chance or represents a finding of significance – are based on probability theory. This is commonly referred to as a p value, the smaller the p value the less likely the possibility that the result has occurred by chance. It is conventionally expressed as $p < 0.05$, though this cut-off is arbitrary (the symbol $<$ identifies it is less than; $>$ would signify more than). Significance levels of 0.05, 0.01 and 0.001 are the most commonly cited p values in relation to significance of findings. A value of 0.05 identifies that the results are significant at a 5 per cent level, meaning that there is less than five chances in a hundred (or 1 in 20) likelihood that the result has occurred by chance. The p value of 0.05 is generally accepted as the level at which it is possible to claim a positive result. There are two commonly used tests to consider significance – chi-squared and t-test:

- The chi-squared test identifies significance between groups.
- The t-test identifies differences between groups.

Where statistical significance is identified, confidence intervals are usually calculated to work out how precise the results are. The wider the interval, the less likely the same results would be found if the research was to be repeated a number of times. If you found that wound dressing X improved wound healing in 65 per cent of the sample, there is a need to know how precise that estimate is if it is to be applied to the wider population. The sample result is unlikely to be exactly the same as the population response to the treatment. It is possible to calculate an interval (with an upper and lower limit) in relation to the sample result that suggests the range within which the target population response to treatment will fall. If the confidence interval had a lower limit of 25 per cent and a higher limit of 100 per cent, the confidence interval is very wide and, therefore, the value of 65 per cent is very imprecise. If, however, the confidence interval is between 60 and 70 per cent, the estimate of 65 per cent is more precise and more meaningful. By convention, researchers usually report confidence intervals of 95 per cent (expressed as 95 per cent CI), which are the range of values (the interval) within which there is 95 per cent confidence that the real value applies to the total population of patients.

Findings

It is usually the norm that descriptive statistics are presented first, to give the readers an overview of the variables. Findings are then generally ordered in terms of importance or in relation to the sequencing of the research question/hypotheses. Tables are used where a number of statistical tests are reported. Tables should be presented in a clear and easily understandable manner, with clear links to the written narrative. All data should be accounted for.

Reliability, validity and applicability

Reliability relates to the accuracy and consistency of findings, whether the same results would be reached if the same variables were repeatedly measured in the same way (Bowling, 2014). For example, you may be fairly sure that a thermometer will accurately measure your temperature and that it would give the same results on repeated measurement at five-minute intervals. If two results varied by five degrees, the reliability of the thermometer would need to be questioned. In critically appraising research, whether the research design, methodology and measurement tools provide accurate findings are being considered and whether, if repeated, the same result would be found.

Validity is described by Polit and Beck (2018) as a property of inference. Researchers can only infer that a perceived effect is a result of their hypothesised case if the research is valid: namely, that there is confidence that what was intended to be measured has been measured. Four types of validity are proposed by Polit and Beck:

1. Statistical conclusion validity – where tests are deemed to be appropriate/fair and any identified statistical relationship between the variables is based on sound evidence.
2. Internal validity – where a relationship is proven that this is the result of the independent variable, not some other circumstance, such as chance, confounding variables, introduction of bias, etc. (see Table 7.3).
3. Construct validity – relates to the degree a tool measures the thing it is designed to measure. For instance, you may be fairly sure that a thermometer is a valid tool to measure temperature (unless it's broken in some way) but you might be less sure of a tool designed to measure pain.
4. External validity – concerns the generalisability of findings to other people and/or settings.

Table 7.4 gives an overview of some of the issues that threaten validity in relation to the above items.

Table 7.3   Sources of bias

Type	Description
Selection bias	Inadequate randomisation or systematic error in the way participants are recruited into a study
Performance bias	Differences in the way intervention is received/delivered
Attrition bias	More subjects are lost from one research group than another (control or experimental)

(Continued)

Table 7.3   (Continued)

Type	Description
Detection bias	Differences which occur when assessing outcomes or RCTs
Participant bias	A lack of full disclosure or giving what is considered to be appropriate responses
Conceptual bias	Faulty conceptualisation of problem, interpretation of findings or drawing of conclusions
Design bias	Faults in any aspect of the research design
Recall bias	Difficulties relating to recalling past events, memory degeneration over time

Validity can also be compromised by confounding variables. As discussed earlier, confounding variables are where a proposed relationship between two variables may actually be due to a third variable. In critically appraising studies you must consider whether the researcher has considered potential confounding variables in the research design and analysis of the findings.

Table 7.4   Factors that may affect validity

Type of validity	Threats to validity
Statistical conclusion	Sample size is small
	Tools lacking the precision to accurately measure the variables
	Variations in the implementation of an intervention
	Treatment adherence
Construct validity	Hawthorne or placebo effect – people's behaviour as a response to being observed or to treatment because they believe it will have a positive effect
	Researcher's response to subjects encourages certain responses
	Novelty effect – perception of new treatments may result in positive or negative responses from subjects
	Compensation – control group subjects are 'compensated' in some way by health staff or family for not receiving research intervention
	Contamination – control and experimental group receive similar services generally or experimental group member moves to control group by dropping out of the trial

Choose and locate a quantitative article of interest and critically appraise it using the questions in Appendix 6. Identify aspects where you need to develop further skills and knowledge. Then develop an action plan outlining how you will develop the knowledge and skills you require to complete the task appropriately.

Activity 7.5

Summary

- The aim of quantitative research is to explore relationships between variables and test hypotheses. The researcher identifies the variables of interest, clearly defines what these are and then collects data, usually in a numerical form.
- The relationships between independent variables and dependent variables are considered. Statistics help in making judgements and generalisations of the value of the research findings for the research population as a whole.
- Two types of research design are present within quantitative research: experimental and non-experimental.
- Quantitative research generally uses what is known as probability sampling.
- There are four levels of measurement within quantitative research – nominal, ordinal, interval and ratio. The level of measurement indicates the statistical test to be used.

FURTHER READING

Bowling, A. (2014) *Research Methods in Health* (4th edn). New York: Open University Press. This book gives a good introduction to research and its use in the healthcare setting.

Carneiro, I (2017) *Introduction to Epidemiology (Understanding Public Health)* (3rd edn). Maidenhead: Open University Press. A very informative book on different approaches to quantitative study design.

Parahoo, K. (2014) *Nursing Research: Principles, Process and Issues* (3rd edn). Basingstoke: Palgrave Macmillan. This is recommended as a guide for beginners but is also useful to those with some research experience.

Saks, M. and Allsop, J. (2012) *Researching Health: Qualitative, Quantitative and Mixed Methods* (2nd edn). London: SAGE Publications. This text offers a wide range of perspectives on health research with a useful and comprehensive section on quantitative methods and health.

Scott, I. and Mazhindu, D. (2014) *Statistics for Health Care Professionals: An Introduction* (2nd edn). London: SAGE Publications.

USEFUL WEBLINKS

CETL Reusable Learning Objects: this website provides reusable learning objects (RLOs) related to a range of topics. These are multimedia overviews of various topics. The 'EBP' and 'Statistics' sections contain RLOs related to the content of this chapter. www.rlo-cetl.ac.uk/index.php

CONSORT website: provides explanations and examples of what is expected to be included in some forms of quantitative research. www.consort-statement.org

Critical Appraisal Skills Programme Checklists: provides a range of checklists to help with critiquing quantitative studies, including tools for systematic reviews, randomised control trials, cohort studies, case control studies, economic evaluations and diagnostic studies. www.casp-uk.net/casp-tools-checklists

Netting the Evidence: www.nettingtheevidence.org.uk

8

Critical Appraisal and Qualitative Research

Janet Barker and Paul Linsley

Learning Outcomes

By the end of the chapter you will be able to:

- discuss qualitative research and its basic traits;
- list qualitative forms of data collection;
- identify the key areas for consideration when critically appraising qualitative literature;
- identify criteria used for evaluating the rigour of qualitative studies.

INTRODUCTION

This chapter considers the methods and approaches used in qualitative research and discusses the issues which should be considered when critically appraising literature of this type. However, as with the previous chapter, it is not the intention to provide a full overview of the research process, and for a more in-depth explanation you need to explore some of the recommended reading at the end of the chapter.

There has been a tendency to equate the idea of 'evidence' with quantitative data produced in the context of experimental or well-controlled quasi-experimental research. Indeed, such research continues to provide the foundation on which health-care policy is built and debated. This situation is being challenged and there is a growing recognition of the importance of qualitative research in informing and shaping clinical practice. Qualitative research has been particularly used in the social sciences – sociology, psychology and anthropology – and many of the healthcare professions – nursing, pharmacy and social work. Furthermore, researchers are increasingly adopting mixed methods in their studies, where qualitative and quantitative approaches are used in combination to address the issues under consideration.

WHAT IS QUALITATIVE RESEARCH?

As discussed in Chapter 2, qualitative research represents a different research paradigm to quantitative research. Qualitative research is a broad term for a variety of research approaches. It has different philosophical underpinnings, which give rise to different ways of thinking about the nature of knowledge and how this can be generated. Whereas positivistic research assumes that phenomena are best understood from an objective standpoint, qualitative research assumes that meaning and knowledge are constructed in a social context (Anfara and Mertz, 2006). As a result of this, many qualitative researchers express a commitment to viewing events in the social world through the eyes of the people that they study. To this end, health and social care are seen as social constructs and their meaning subject to changes in social norms across time and geographical areas. Qualitative research employs methods that reflect and in part capture the complexities of the topic and the real world in which events are played out. The researcher attempts to understand the person's worldview through a variety of methods and focuses on the interpretation of words; how people describe their experiences, perspectives, understanding, beliefs and values. The words collected may be in spoken or written form.

Qualitative research is an attempt to provide what is termed as a **rich** or **thick description** of the phenomenon from an **emic** (individual's) perspective rather than an **etic** (outsider's, or researcher's) perspective: namely, to give a full and thorough account of the research context, the meanings people attach to their experiences, their interpretation of issues and also what motivates them to behave/respond in particular ways. Qualitative research is seen as being holistic, giving a total picture of a phenomenon rather than considering parts in isolation. In short, qualitative research is concerned with the social aspects of our world and often seeks to find answers to the following questions (Parahoo, 2014):

- Why do people behave the way they do?
- How are opinions and attitudes formed?
- How are people affected by the events that go on around them?
- How and why have cultures developed in the way they have?
- What are the differences between social groups or between males and females?

It is suggested that qualitative research has six central traits (see Table 8.1) (Streubert and Carpenter, 2010).

Table 8.1   Six basic traits of qualitative research

Trait	Description
Belief in multiple realities	There is no one reality/truth
	People actively construct their understanding of the world
	People have different experiences of life
	A number of perspectives are available in relation to any situation/phenomenon
An understanding of the nature of the phenomena being studied through appropriate methods is provided	There are multiple ways of understanding various phenomena
	The most appropriate approach(es) to 'capturing' these understandings must be used
	The phenomenon under consideration dictates the method to be used
	Multiple forms of data collection are often used to ensure a full understanding of the research topic
Provides an understanding from the subject/ participant's point of view	Qualitative research involves developing a theory in relation to a phenomenon – asking questions such as 'what do you experience of caring?' from someone with a learning disability
Research is conducted in the natural environment in which the phenomenon occurs	No attempt is made to control the environment
	The natural environment provides a way of accessing the participant's perspective whilst in the 'space' that it occurs
	Gives access to any cues or influences on the individual's perspective
The researcher as part of the process	Acceptance that all research is conducted in a subjective way
	Researcher is seen as adding to the richness of the data
Data are said to be 'rich' and 'deep'	Data are collected in the form of words, describing the perspectives and experiences of the participants

TYPES OF QUALITATIVE RESEARCH

There a number of approaches to qualitative research, each with their own theoretical and philosophical underpinnings. The most common approaches are outlined below, and an overview of their various aspects is presented in Table 8.2.

Phenomenology

This approach is based in a philosophical tradition developed by Edmund Husserl (1857–1938) and Martin Heidegger (1889–1976), which considers people's everyday experiences. The focus here is to explore the meaning that people attach to their lived experience and is closely related to **hermeneutics**, which centres on meaning and interpretation – how people interpret their experiences within a specific context. For example, if you wanted to know what it means to someone to be given a diagnosis of cancer, how they experience this, you might undertake a phenomenological study.

Key question: What are the meaning, structure and essence of the lived experience of this phenomenon by an individual(s)?

Grounded theory

Developed by sociologists Glaser and Strauss (1967), grounded theory is an approach origi-nally forwarded as a way of developing theories and hypotheses that are 'grounded' in the data collected. Strauss and Corbin (1990: 7) describe a grounded theory as one that 'is discovered, developed, and provisionally verified through systematic data collection and analysis of data pertaining to the phenomenon'. It is based on the idea that human behaviour is developed through people's interactions and their interpretation of these. It is often used to study social processes, considering the changes that occur over time in relation to particular experiences. In nursing it is frequently used to gain an understanding of the process through which people learn to manage and/or adapt to a new situation. For example, this approach could be used to consider how children adapt their lives over time following a diagnosis of diabetes.

Key question: What theory or explanation emerges from an analysis of the data collected about this phenomenon?

Ethnography

This research approach has its roots in anthropology, being used to consider beliefs, values and shared meanings of people in particular cultures. Leininger (1985: 35) defined eth-nography as 'the systematic process of observing, detailing, describing, documenting and analysing the lifeways or particular patterns of a culture (or subculture)'. Cultures in this context could relate to an entire social group (such as the culture of people from Romania) or to a small group (such as a particular ward setting). Therefore, you could study the beliefs and values of people from Romania in relation to the care of people with learning disabilities. Alternatively, you could study how the culture of a particular residential home for people with learning disabilities impacts on the care given.

Key question: What are the cultural characteristics of this group of people or this cultural setting?

Action research

Action research can include both qualitative and quantitative approaches and is used to study the effects of actions when these are taken to change or improve something. There are various forms of action research, but the basic tenet is that it is a group activity (Streubert and Carpenter, 2010), usually involving some form of collaboration between the researcher and the partici-pants – practitioners, patients or other stakeholders in the process – with a view to improving/ changing practices in a specific area. It is also said to be context bound, in that the research is undertaken because of a defined issue related to a specific area. Its participants are seen as central to decision-making processes and have the final say as to whether changes are implemented or not. It is often seen as cyclic in nature, with problems being identified, changes made and impact evaluated. For instance, this approach could be used to consider the most appropriate way to change how 'clinical handover' is organised in a particular ward setting.

Key question: What have we learnt from implementing this change?

Discourse analysis

Discourse analysis is relatively new to nursing research and looks at the ways in which people talk about particular issues; for example, the systems people use in communicating with each other. It tries to uncover the rules that govern how people talk about things. Its basic premise is that language is not neutral: when talking, what is said and how it is said has particular meaning and intentions. Foucault's (1979) work has been particularly influential in this area, focusing on how power is exercised through the use of language. For example, it would be possible to consider what power relations are present when qualified nurses talk to students and what values are present in the language they use.

Key question: How is the information presented and whose interest does it serve?

Historical research

As a research approach, historical methods collect and interpret historical data in a system-atic way. The aim is to provide new insights into a topic area, not to summarise existing knowledge as might be done with a literature review (Streubert and Carpenter, 2010). Generally, the form of historical research is underpinned by a particular theoretical frame-work, such as feminism or postmodernism. Historical research may be in the form of biographical accounts of individuals who provide oral histories of particular groups; for example, oral histories could be taken from people who have experienced mental health institutions at various points in the twentieth century.

Key question: What can we learn from what has gone before?

Case study

Another popular form of qualitative research is the use of a case study. A case study refers to an in-depth analysis of a single person, a group of people, an organisation or an institution, often as a series of vignettes. Case studies can be quite complex in their design and track a person or series of events over time. According to Yin (2018) a case study design should be considered when: (a) the focus of the study is to answer 'how' and 'why' questions; (b) you cannot manipulate the behaviour of those involved in the study; (c) you want to cover contextual conditions because you believe they are relevant to the phenomenon under study; or (d) the boundaries are not clear between the phenomenon and context.

Key question: What is happening or has happened? How or why did something happen the way it did?

While the relationships between theory and qualitative methods may appear complex they provide the 'scaffolding' (Anfara and Mertz, 2006) from which researchers go about constructing and conducting their studies. Furthermore, while qualitative researchers will claim to use a particular approach to their study, it is not unusual to see a combining of data collection methods; for example, case study data may be used and analysed using grounded theory. One of the strengths of qualitative research is its responsiveness to a changing situation and its ability to pursue new lines of enquiry as they emerge.

Activity 8.1

Find one piece of research for each of the research approaches identified in Table 8.2 relevant to your own field of practice. Consider how each piece might inform your practice and how it shapes your understanding of the topic under investigation.

Table 8.2   Overview of qualitative research approaches

Approach	Types of research questions	Data collection	Example
Phenomenology	Meaning/lived experience	Unstructured interviews	Freeman, L., Fothergill-Bourbonnais, F. and Rashotte, J. (2014) The experience of being a trauma nurse: A phenomenological study. *Intensive and Critical Care Nursing*, 30, 1, 6–12.
Grounded theory	Social settings Process questions	Interviews Observation	Sadeghi, T., Nayeri ,N. D. and Abbaszadeh, A. (2015) The waiting process: A grounded theory study of families' experiences of waiting for patients during surgery. *Journal of Research in Nursing*, 20, 5, 372–382.
Ethnography	Culture Beliefs and values	Participant observation Field notes Interviews	Dupin, C.M., Borglin, G., Debout, C. and Rothan-Tondeur, M. (2014) An ethnographic study of nurses' experience with nursing research and its integration into practice. *Journal of Advanced Nursing*, 70, 9, 2128–2139.
Discourse analysis	Verbal interaction What power relationships are present in conversations?	Observation Recording of interactions Field notes	Yazdannik, A., Yousefy, A. and Mohammadi, S. (2017) Discourse analysis: A useful methodology for health care system researches. *Journal of Education and Health Promotion*, 6: 111, published online www.ncbi.nlm.nih.gov/pmc/articles/ PMC5747223/

Approach	Types of research questions	Data collection	Example
Action research	Implementing change	Mixed	Parker, V., Lieschke, G. and Giles, M. (2017) Ground-up-top down: A mixed method action research study aimed at normalising research in practice for nurses and midwives. *BMC Nursing*, BMC series, 16:52, published online https://bmcnurs. biomedcentral.com/articles/10.1186/ s12912-017-0249-8#Abs1
Historical	Identifying historical roots and/or practices	Interviews Narratives Documentation	Dunne, B., Pettigrew, J. and Robinson, K. (2015) Using historical documentary methods to explore the history of occupational therapy. *British Journal of Occupational Therapy*, 79, 6, 376–384.
Case study	How or why a thing happened the way it did	Analysis of an event presented as a written account or presentation	Shaban, R.Z., Considine, J., Fry, M. and Curtis, K. (2017) Case study and case-based research in emergency nursing and care: Theoretical foundations and practical application in paramedic pre-hospital clinical judgement and decision-making of patients with mental illness. *Australian Emergency Nursing Journal*, 20, 17–24.

CRITICAL APPRAISAL

As discussed in relation to quantitative research, a number of tools are available to help with critical appraisal research, of which many are specifically aimed at qualitative research (Caldwell et al., 2005). The first tool, CASP, helps evaluate studies in journals. The criteria that follow this offer a more rigorous standard for the construction, reporting and review of both qualitative and quantitative research. Appendix 7 gives a generic approach to this form of critique, and those areas specific to qualitative research are highlighted and discussed below in conjunction with those shared with quantitative research as discussed in Chapter 6. Again, as identified previously, have good research books to hand so information can be checked or clarified along the way.

- *Critical Appraisal Tools for the Evaluation of Published Studies* Called the CASP (Critical Appraisal Skills Programme) Tools of the Public Health Research Unit of the National Health Service (UK), it contains separate study evaluation tools for systematic reviews, randomised control trials, economic evaluation studies, qualitative studies, cohort studies, case control studies and diagnostic test studies (see www.casp–uk.net).

- *COREQ (Consolidated criteria for reporting qualitative research)* (see http://intqhc.oxford journals.org/content/19/6/349).
- *STROBE (Strengthening the Reporting of Observational Studies)* For use with observational studies, case–control and cross–sectional studies (see www.strobe-statement.org/Checklist.html).
- *CONSORT (Consolidated Standards of Reporting Trials)* For randomised control trials (RCTs) (see www.consort-statement.org).
- *STARD (Standards of Reporting Diagnostic Accuracy)* For diagnostic test studies (see www.stard-statement.org).
- *AMSTAR* A measurement tool to assess systematic reviews (see www.pubmedcentral.nih.gov/articlerender.fcgi?artid=2131785).
- *MOOSE (Meta-Analyses of Observational Studies in Epidemiology)* (see www.editorial manager.com/jognn/account/MOOSE.pdf).
- *WHO Minimal Registration Data Set for Clinical Trials Registry Recommendations* (see www.who.int/ictrp/network/trds/en).
- *Equator Network* is a Resource Centre for improving research reporting, ethics and dissemination of publishing standards, as well as posting reporting criteria (see www.equator-network.org/?o=1028#guidance).

A number of sites offer critical appraisal tools and remind us how to classify the types of study and rank the hierarchy or levels of evidence they produce. The Centre for Evidence-Based Medicine at Oxford was the first established for this purpose (see www.cebm.net).

Activity 8.2

Take time out to explore each of the above sites. Make a note of what you found useful and when you might call on this as part of your clinical work.

Research question and aims

Qualitative research normally will have a research question and not a hypothesis, as the intention is to generate understanding in relation to a phenomenon not to predict a relationship between variables. The research question can take two forms (Cormack, Gerrish and Lathlean 2015):

1. Interrogative – namely, a statement phrased as a question, e.g. 'What is the lived experience of people admitted to hospital following a suicide attempt?'

2. Declarative – namely, a statement which 'declares' the purpose of the study, e.g. 'It is intended to study the experience of people admitted to hospital following a suicide attempt.'

The best research questions are short and clearly identify a specific area of study. The question should set the scene for the research design that will allow the question to be answered. Some researchers will pose a series of questions while others identify a series of aims in relation to the question asked. The research question and aims should have the same intentions.

Literature review

An extensive literature review is not always the starting point of qualitative research. Often, only sufficient literature to provide a focus for the study will be considered. In phenomenological research the literature may not be reviewed until after the data have been collected and analysed. In grounded theory the literature is reviewed at various points throughout the data collection process and is used as a comparison for the interim research findings. This lack of initial literature review is to ensure that the analysis of the data is not influenced by what is already known about the topic. However, there is an expectation that the findings will be considered in light of the available literature, so that the study can be compared with other work and any issues regarding the **transferability** of findings to other settings can be identified.

Where a literature review is provided, the criteria identified by Parahoo (2014) described in Chapter 6 (see p. 99) can be applied.

Methodology

The chosen methodology should enable the research question to be answered. If the question asks about the meaning of something or an individual's experience, then you would expect to see a phenomenological design. If the stated aim is to investigate issues related to culture – beliefs, values, social norms – then an ethnographic approach would be more appropriate. There should be a match between what the researcher wants to know and the methodology used to answer the question. Table 8.2 gives an idea of the methodologies expected to be seen in relation to particular areas of study.

Reflexivity

While researcher involvement in the research process is a central tenet of qualitative research, there is also an expectation that researchers will discuss their beliefs, values, ideas and personal biases relating to the topic they are exploring, and this is usually given in the form of a reflective account. This reflexivity is seen as having two purposes. First, it makes the investigators aware of how their own beliefs may influence the data collection and interpretation. Having explored their own perspectives it is normally expected that researchers will put aside their beliefs in what is termed as **bracketing**. Here researchers are expected not to make judgements about the appropriateness of what they see or hear, instead being open to what the data reveal rather than imposing their own beliefs on it. The second aspect relates to acknowledging that the researcher is part of the research process and ensures that the reader is aware of this.

Activity 8.3

Identify an area you would be interested in researching. Write a short reflective piece identifying what beliefs and values you have in relation to the area and how that might impact on any research you undertook.

However, while this process is an integral part of qualitative research, often the reflective account is missing from published work. The word limits imposed by journal publishers on authors of papers frequently result in this aspect being left out. When this is the case, the only insight given into the researchers' perspectives and backgrounds in terms of the research phenomenon is gained through examining their qualifications and job titles given at the beginning of the article.

Ethical issues

As identified in Chapter 6, all health service research requires ethical approval; however, the nature of qualitative research brings a distinct set of ethical issues into view. The interpersonal nature of most qualitative research (i.e. that the researcher and participants are in direct contact and form a close, albeit brief, trusting relationship) requires the researcher to be aware of any possible emotional impact the research may have on participants. Streubert and Carpenter (2010) identify various aspects that are important in qualitative research, and these are areas you should consider when doing a critical appraisal:

1. Informed consent – within qualitative research participants must be allowed to withdraw this consent at any point. 'Process informed' consent is often adopted, where a participant's consent will be re-evaluated at various points within the study and involvement stopped if required.
2. Confidentiality and anonymity – the one-to-one interaction between participant and researcher means that anonymity is not possible in the same way as in quantitative research; the researcher will obviously know where the data came from. However, confidentiality can and must be maintained, with every effort made to ensure that participants are not recognisable in the data used to support descriptions of results.
3. The researcher–participant relationship – the researcher must be clear about the boundaries of this relationship. This is a particular issue for healthcare professionals, who may find their role as care provider conflicting with their role of researcher.
4. Sensitive issues – some of the issues discussed during data collection can be distressing for the participants and/or the researcher. It is important that the researcher identifies

mechanisms for dealing with such issues and how participants will be supported following data collection.

> Imagine you are conducting a research study discussing a topic which may cause the participants to become distressed. What support do you think it would be important to offer to the participants?
>
> **Activity 8.4**

Sampling/participant selection

Individuals are usually selected to participate in particular research because they will have had experience of or are involved in the phenomenon being studied. For instance, if the research question is 'What is the lived experience of people with schizophrenia?' the people selected to participate in the study would be people with schizophrenia, as only they would be able to describe their experiences.

As the intention with qualitative research is to gain a greater understanding of the area of interest, not to generalise findings, randomised sampling is not an issue here. There are various approaches to sampling the population of interest:

- Convenience – the most conveniently available people are selected, those who are closest to hand and relevant to the phenomenon of interest.
- Snowballing – a form of convenience sampling where having identified an informant to tell you about the phenomenon, they then identify someone else.
- Purposive or purposeful – selecting people who can tell you about the research phenomenon; this approach tends to be used in phenomenological studies.
- Theoretical – a framework is created in which the principal concepts related to the study are identified and individuals are selected to participate who are judged to have theoretical purpose/relevance; the researcher clearly states the basic types of participants to be included and how these individuals will facilitate the collection of appropriate data to describe the phenomenon. This approach is most often seen in grounded theory.

Sample sizes in qualitative research are normally small in comparison to quantitative research. It is not unusual to see research conducted on just 10 people. The nature of the data collected and subsequent analysis makes large samples almost impossible to handle. For example, one 45-minute interview can produce 30 pages of transcribed information. Just 10 participants would therefore result in around 300 pages requiring analysis. The aim of qualitative research is to reduce this huge amount of information to a manageable size without losing the participants' intended meaning.

The sample size is largely decided by the type of research, the quality of the information provided by the participants and the sampling approach used. Often, qualitative researchers talk about reaching **data saturation**, particularly in grounded theory. This is the point where no new information is being collected from participants and is usually the point where data collection stops. So, for example, if data saturation is reached after interviewing 12 people then no further interviews will be conducted.

Data collection

There are various forms of data collection available to the qualitative researcher, but most involve the collection of 'words' in some shape or form. Table 8.3 provides an overview of the main types of activity. In appraising a study it is important to consider whether the form of data collection used will provide the researcher with the most appropriate data.

It is essential that a study identifies how the information from participants was recorded. Many researchers will use audio recording devices, some may incorporate video recording to ensure that non-verbal responses are captured. While field notes are useful and add to the picture, they tend to be incomplete and do not enable the researcher to revisit the interaction in its original form. Remember, these data collection methods are often used to gain an understanding of persons' or populations':

- attitudes
- behaviours
- value systems
- concerns
- motivations
- aspirations
- culture
- lifestyles

Table 8.3   Types of data collection

Type	Description
Interviews	Unstructured – no prepared questions apart from asking them to talk about the phenomenon of interest
	Semi-structured – a guide asking open questions related to the areas of interest, prepared in advance
	(Structured – not used in qualitative research)
Focus groups	Group interviews, 6–12 people discussing a topic
Observation	Participant observation – the researcher is part of the group and is involved in its activities
	Observer-participant – the researcher generally observes and may interview members of the group and may also participate in some activities
	Complete observer – no interaction between observer and participant
Field notes	In ethnography these involve documenting observations and narratives
	In phenomenology these may involve recording individual expressions and other aspects not captured by audio recording of interviews

Type	Description
Diaries	Unstructured – where people are asked simply to record their thoughts and feelings
	Structured – where people are asked to write about specific aspects
Documentation	Patient notes, historical records, health service documentation and records; published and unpublished works

Data analysis

Polit and Beck (2018) propose that qualitative data analysis is more difficult to do than quantitative analysis but easier to understand, which is a bonus for those who are critiquing rather than doing the research. However, it is not always easy to fully appraise the findings, as you cannot know if the authors have given an appropriate representation of participants' narratives.

Qualitative analysis usually involves some sort of content analysis where researchers create categories and themes from the data. As these categories are created, a coding system is then developed which allows statements made by participants to be grouped together in particular categories. Once such categories have been identified these may then be further grouped into themes. Data can be handled manually or analysed using computer-assisted qualitative data analysis systems (CAQDAS) such as NVivo. However, as there are a number of approaches to qualitative research, the content analysis takes various forms. Note this lack of a universal approach can make it difficult to critically appraise the work.

When critically appraising a qualitative analysis you are looking to see whether the author has given you enough information to make a judgement as to whether the analysis has been conducted in an appropriate way. There are a number of basic tenets you would expect to be described:

1. Data transcription – how the data are translated from audio to a written form; what steps were taken to ensure data were of the best quality, including identification of problems related to transcription (e.g. background noise, poor tape quality, participant's voice inaudible).
2. Identification of tool used for analysis – a number of tools would be available and the one chosen should be appropriate to the research methodology. For example, you would not expect a grounded theory methodology to include Colaizzi's (1978) approach, which is specific to phenomenology. The researcher involved should clearly identify the approach taken and you should be able to follow this step-by-step through the paper.
3. Interpretation – this occurs at the same time as the analysis, as the researcher reads and re-reads the data and the codes, categories/themes and tries to make sense of the data. The writer should give details of how the interpretation was arrived at.

Throughout the course of qualitative analysis, the analyst should be asking and re-asking the following questions:

- What patterns and common themes emerge in responses dealing with specific items? How do these patterns (or lack thereof) help to illuminate the broader study question(s)?
- Are there any deviations from these patterns? If yes, are there any factors that might explain these atypical responses?
- What interesting stories emerge from the responses? How can these stories help to illuminate the broader study question(s)?
- Do any of these patterns or findings suggest that additional data may need to be collected? Do any of the study questions need to be revised?
- Do the patterns that emerge corroborate the findings of any corresponding qualitative analyses that have been conducted? If not, what might explain these discrepancies?

Activity 8.5

Find three different examples of tools that can be used in the analysis of qualitative data.

Issues of rigour

Streubert and Carpenter (2010) suggested that decisions as to the **rigour** of a particular research study are a 'judgement call'. They go on to suggest that two fundamental characteristics of qualitative research should be present when making this judgement as to whether it meets the implicit goal of providing an accurate account of participants' perspective:

1. Is there adequate attention to the collection of information?
2. Is there confirmation of the accuracy of the information?

Table 8.4   Criteria for assessing rigour of qualitative research

Criteria	Ways of identifying if criteria are met
Credibility	Findings returned to participants for confirmation that they are a true representation of their experiences
	All data are accounted for, including instances where the data are inconsistent with other findings
	Triangulation
Dependability	Reporting of unexpected events and how dealt with
	Recording methods ensured quality of data
	Triangulation

Criteria	Ways of identifying if criteria are met
Confirmability	Evidence of reflexivity
	Provision of an 'audit trail' to enable the thought and decision-making processes to be identified (a research diary or recording mechanisms within CAQDAS)
Transferability	Providing a full description of the research setting and participants
	Identifying that the findings have relevance to similar situations
	Theoretical triangulation
Authenticity	The reality of the participants' lives is conveyed, enabling you to understand the range of feelings experienced by those involved

MIXED METHODOLOGY

Mixed methodology, or **triangulation** as it is otherwise called, is broadly defined as the combination of methodologies in a study of the same phenomenon. A mixed method approach is considered as having been adopted where the mixing of methods occurs within paradigms, sampling, data collection or analytic techniques (Green and Thorogood, 2018). Mixed methodology of this kind is philosophically congruent with the view that research paradigms exist upon a continuum rather than being competitively divergent (O'Byrne, 2007). The strength of such an approach is that the same issue can be explored from different and consequently fuller perspectives, offering a greater understanding of the phenomena under investigation (Wuest, 2011). Each data collection method used represents one stage of a larger process.

Four types of triangulation are possible (Denzin, 2017):

1. Data triangulation – where more than one source of data is collected. This can be done in three ways:
   a. Time – collecting data at different points in time: for instance, you might interview people at intervals of three, six and twelve months in relation to a particular phenomenon.
   b. Space – collecting data from different sites: for example, including different in-patient units in a study.
   c. Person – collecting information from different groups of people: for example, interviewing nurses on band 5, 6 and 7; or service users and their carers.
2. Methodological triangulation – two or more research methods are used in:
   d. The research design – for example, combining qualitative and quantitative approaches.
   e. The data collection techniques – for example, using diaries and interviews.

3. Investigator triangulation – here two or more investigators, each having their own specific area of expertise, will collect, analyse and interpret the data.
4. Theoretical triangulation – having more than one theory underpinning the analysis of the data. As the data are analysed they are viewed through the 'lens' of different theories to see if alternative interpretations arise from examining them in multiple ways.

Activity 8.6

What would you take into consideration in determining whether the study you are reading is a qualitative, quantitative or mixed methods research? What are the characteristics of each?

Activity 8.7

Choose one of the research articles identified in Table 8.2 and critically appraise it using the questions in Appendix 7. Identify the aspects/questions where you need to develop further skills and knowledge. Develop an action plan outlining how you will develop the knowledge and skills you require to complete the task appropriately.

Summary

- There are a number of approaches to qualitative research, each with their own theoretical and philosophical underpinning, generally focusing on how people describe their experiences, perspectives, understanding and beliefs/values.
- Ethical issues take a particular form in qualitative research.
- Sample sizes in qualitative research are normally small in comparison to quantitative research. Individuals are usually invited to participate in particular research because they have experience or are involved in the phenomenon being studied.
- There are various forms of data collection available to the qualitative researcher, but most of them involve the collecting of 'words' in some shape or form and analysis involves some sort of content analysis where the researcher creates categories and themes from the data.

FURTHER READING

Green, J. and Thorogood, N. (2014) *Qualitative Methods for Health Research*. London: Sage.

Polit, D.F. and Beck, C.T. (2016) *Nursing Research: Generating and Assessing Evidence for Nursing Practice* (10th edn). Philadelphia: Lippincott Williams and Wilkins. This book gives a good introduction to the various aspects of qualitative research and its approaches.

Streubert, H.J. and Carpenter, D.R. (2010) *Qualitative Research in Nursing. Advancing the Humanistic Imperative* (5th edn). Philadelphia: Lippincott Williams and Wilkins. This provides an overview of various aspects of qualitative research, the different approaches and guidelines, to help in the critical appraisal of the different methods.

USEFUL WEBLINKS

Critical Appraisal Skills Programme: provides a range of resources to help with developing the skills associated with EBP. Also provides a range of critical appraisal tools. www.casp-uk.net

QualPage: provides resources and information related to qualitative research. The methods section provides an overview of different qualitative methodologies. www.qualitativeresearch.uga.edu/QualPage

Netting the Evidence: Google Search Engine – searches 107 sites associated with EBP. http://tinyurl.com/2poh3a

9

Systematic Reviews and Evidence-based Practice

Marishona Ortega and Janet Barker

Learning Outcomes

By the end of the chapter you will be able to:

- discuss the systematic review process and its key features;
- identify key areas for consideration when critically appraising systematic reviews;
- identify issues to be considered when assessing the rigour of systematic reviews.

INTRODUCTION

> The notion of systematic review – looking at the totality of evidence – is quietly one of the most important innovations in medicine over the past 30 years. (Goldacre, 2011)

The explosion of literature related to healthcare has made it almost impossible for any practitioner to keep abreast of all current research findings. As has already been mentioned in Chapter 5, the US National Library of Medicine added more than 800,000 citations to

Medline in 2017 alone (US National Library of Medicine, 2018). It has even been estimated that by 2020, it will only take 73 days for medical knowledge to double (Densen, 2011).

As identified in Chapter 1, in many ways EBP is seen as having its origins in Professor Archie Cochrane's criticisms of the medical profession for its failure to use the body of evidence available to it in an appropriate way and his call for the development of up to date 'critical summaries' of all randomised control trials (RCTs) relevant to a specialty or sub-specialty (Cochrane, 1979). This ultimately led to the formation of the Cochrane Collaboration in 1993 and the Cochrane Database of Systematic Reviews in 1995. Prior to the emergence of EBP, summaries of studies more frequently appeared in the form of what Greenhalgh (2014) terms as 'journalistic reviews'. Here papers were reviewed, selected and analysed in an ad hoc manner, subject to the vagaries of the person conducting the literature review. In many ways this left any interpretation provided open to accusations of bias, and the lack of a systematic approach gave the reader little evidence on which to consider the credibility of the findings. However, since the advent of EBP, systematic reviews have become more prevalent; between its launch in 2011 and the end of 2017, 30,000 systematic reviews were registered on PROSPERO, the international database of prospectively registered systematic reviews in health and social care (Page et al., 2018). Although systematic reviews employ rigorous methods, which are explicit and reproducible, critical appraisal of systematic reviews is just as important as appraising single studies before implementing any results into your practice.

This chapter will consider the methods and approaches used in systematic reviews and the areas to be considered when critically appraising this form of evidence.

WHAT IS A SYSTEMATIC REVIEW?

Systematic reviews provide a rigorous review of research findings in relation to a specific question, saving nurses and other healthcare professionals the time and effort it would take to search and appraise a large body of evidence in order to keep up to date with knowledge in their field. Systematic reviews are also often used as a starting point for the development of clinical practice guidelines and protocols (Moher et al. 2009; Tonin et al., 2017). Parahoo defines systematic reviews as 'the rigorous and systematic search, selection, appraisal, synthesis and summary of the findings of primary research studies in order to answer a specific question' (2014: 123). While it is not expected that health professionals in general undertake systematic reviews (they can be both complex and time consuming to complete) there is a need to be able to recognise, appraise and evaluate their usefulness for practice.

Systematic reviews are fundamental to EBP, as can be seen in the Evidence Based Health Care (EBHC) Pyramid 5.0 (Alper and Haynes, 2016), where they form one of the levels of sound evidence on which nurses and other healthcare professionals can base practice. Greenhalgh (2014) lists a number of advantages that systematic reviews have over single studies, including the fact that they allow practitioners to assimilate large amounts of information quickly, which speeds up the decision-making process.

Systematic review is a term that is often used interchangeably with **meta-analysis**, but as you will see from the discussion below the two are not the same. Systematic reviews have previously been primarily associated with quantitative research, but systematic reviews of qualitative research with an accompanying **meta–synthesis** of the qualitative findings are becoming increasingly common. Methods for qualitative systematic reviews are still developing, with the Cochrane Database only publishing their first qualitative review in 2013 in what was described as a milestone for the organisation (Gülmezoglu et al., 2013). There are also systematic reviews that use a **mixed methods** approach in which both qualitative and quantitative studies are considered, with both a meta–analysis and meta–synthesis of relevant studies being provided, although this approach is still very much in its infancy (Joanna Briggs Institute, 2014: 6). One advantage of mixed methods reviews is that by maximising their findings they have a greater ability to inform both policy and practice (Pearson et al., 2015).

Following concerns raised about the clarity of reporting in systematic reviews (Moher et al., 2009), guidelines in the form of the PRISMA (Preferred Reporting Items for Systematic Reviews and Meta–Analyses) statement were developed as 'an evidence-based minimum set of items for reporting in systematic reviews and meta–analyses' (PRISMA, 2015a). The PRISMA statement is endorsed by Cochrane and the Centre for Reviews and Dissemination as well as several hundred journals which publish systematic reviews.

Activity 9.1

Visit the PRISMA website (www.prisma-statement.org). Identify two of the items on the checklist provided in relation to a systematic review or meta-analysis that you would like to learn more about. Create an action plan on how you will develop your learning in relation to these two areas. Please note that the PRISMA statement is in the process of being updated to take into account various methodological developments that have taken place in the last decade.

Systematic reviews are a form of research, often termed **secondary research** in that they are based on research already undertaken; however, their strength lies in their ability to reduce potential bias, and improve the reliability and accuracy of conclusions (Akobeng, 2005). Cochrane produce systematic reviews, which are widely recognised as the gold standard, where they 'seek to collate all evidence that fits pre-specified eligibility criteria in order to address a specific research question' (Green et al., 2011). The process of 'collating' this evidence is a systematic process – Box 9.1 identifies the steps associated with systematic reviews.

TYPES OF SYSTEMATIC REVIEWS

There are two main types of systematic review – quantitative and qualitative. The basic steps of each are the same; however, differences occur when analysing and summarising the evidence. While in both types of systematic review the reviewer is 'pooling' the results from 'like' studies and creating a larger data set for analysis (Pearson et al., 2007: 92), the underpinning philosophies and methods used are different. The pooling of quantitative data (meta–analysis) is seen as an aggregation of the findings; the pooling of qualitative findings (meta–synthesis) can be an aggregation or interpretation of findings depending on the approach used. A meta–analysis can also be seen as giving an overall picture of the effectiveness of an intervention, while meta–synthesis increases understanding of a phenomenon of interest. The key features of systematic reviews, whether quantitative or qualitative, are that they are explicit in their methods and statement of objectives and that the methodology employed is transparent and reproducible (Greenhalgh, 2014: 116).

Box 9.1   Systematic review process

1. Formulate and frame question
2. Search for and select relevant literature
3. Assess the quality of the literature
4. Summarise and present findings
5. Conclude and make recommendations

Formulate and frame question

The development of a review protocol should be the first step when undertaking a systematic review. The protocol gives direction and it should describe the rationale, hypothesis and methodology of the planned review. There are various checklists available to facilitate the reporting of protocols, with one example being PRISMA-P (PRISMA, 2015b). In many instances, the protocols of systematic reviews are registered and published, which can help reduce duplication; for example, the protocols for all Cochrane reviews are made available via the Cochrane Database of Systematic Reviews (CDSR) at www.cochranelibrary.com.

All systematic reviews should have a clearly identifiable and well-formulated question; this is sometimes presented in the PICO format or a variation of this. Without this the reviewer and the reader will not be able to decide whether relevant papers are included. While a particular question such as 'Does eating breakfast improve cognitive functioning in children?' may initially sound appropriate, when you start to pull it apart and consider each aspect, such as what is meant by children (all under–18s or a specific group?), breakfast (a slice of toast or a 'full English'?) and cognitive functioning (alertness, memory, understanding, completion of tests?), then it becomes apparent that the need for clear identification of the various aspects is key to the whole process.

As with any research, the objectives should be clearly stated and flow from the question. The inclusion/exclusion criteria identify the limits of the review and give a clear indication of what is to be included in the review and what is not. Sound justifications are expected to be present for the setting of the limits as well as a clear exploration of the implications of these for the review.

Search for and select relevant literature

The methods used to identify the literature relevant to a particular systematic review are a fundamental issue when assessing its rigour. As Pearson et al. (2007: 60) have pointed out, the quality of a systematic review is reduced if the search strategy is poorly designed and implemented. When undertaking a review, the reviewers must ensure that all studies relevant to the topic are identified. This will require the creation of a comprehensive search strategy, which is highly sensitive, thus ensuring that any literature relevant to the review is retrieved. As the validity of the review is reliant on the quality of the search strategy, it is essential that it is clearly reported in the final review. The same principles discussed in Chapter 5 apply when identifying what search terms and databases are appropriate.

According to Booth et al. (2016) the search methods that should be employed in a systematic review are:

- database searching;
- hand searching of journals;
- bibliographic searching such as checking reference lists for potential sources or citation searching;
- searching for grey literature;
- identifying ongoing research;
- contacting experts.

When critically appraising a systematic review, it is important to consider whether all relevant sources of literature have been included as this may have an impact on the rigour of the review.

Activity 9.2

List databases and other sources of information you would consider key to finding literature related to your own area of practice.

Assessing the quality of the literature

The quality of the literature to be included in a systematic review should be assessed and some form of appraisal of each study should be undertaken. Consideration should be given to 'the extent to which its design, conduct, analysis and presentation were appropriate to answer its research question' (Higgins et al., 2011). Study design is often used as a 'general marker of study quality' (Khan et al., 2011: 39); for example, Cochrane systematic reviews will generally only include RCTs. Therefore, only studies meeting a minimum standard will be considered for inclusion.

Consideration must also be given as to what measures have been taken to minimise bias. A bias as defined by the Cochrane Bias Methods Group is 'a systematic error, or deviation from the truth, in results or inferences' (2018). There is a range of tools including scales and checklists available to help identify the potential for bias; alternatively, Cochrane's Risk of Bias Tool (Higgins et al., 2011), can be used to critically assess six domains including selection, performance, detection, attrition, reporting and other forms of bias. Whichever method is employed should be identified and appropriate to the type of research under consideration.

The use of at least two reviewers is also the norm in systematic reviews. They should independently review each study identified and reach agreement as to their eligibility for inclusion in the review. All steps in this process should be transparent and recorded.

Summarise and present findings

The method of summarising the evidence or data extraction should be clearly identified. The purpose of data extraction is to extract the findings from each study in a consistent manner in order to facilitate synthesis. The methods will vary depending on the purpose of the review, but it is important that it is undertaken in as reliable and unbiased a way as possible. There are different types of software available to assist with these processes (see Table 9.1). For quantitative reviews, information about the studies is usually presented in the form of tables identifying:

- study characteristics, e.g. aims, objectives, inclusion and exclusion criteria;
- participant characteristics, e.g. age, gender, ethnicity;
- intervention – details of the exact form of intervention (and control) and how it was delivered (e.g. routes, dosages, timing, instructions for delivery);
- outcome measures – the reviewers should clearly identify what outcome measures are under consideration;
- results of study analysis.

In relation to qualitative reviews it is expected that a study's methodology (phenomenology, ethnography, etc.), cultural features (age, socioeconomic group and ethnicity) and form of data collection (interview, focus group, etc.) will be clearly recorded.

These tables will allow you to compare various studies and help you to make a judgement as to the rigour of the systematic review. If a table indicates there is significant heterogeneity within the studies, then it is unlikely that the results will be subjected to meta-analysis. It is possible to conduct a meta-synthesis of heterogeneous qualitative studies and this is discussed later in the chapter. Where it is not possible or appropriate to pool data in the form of a meta-analysis, a narrative integration or written summary of findings should be provided.

Conclude and make recommendations

The reviewers should justify their conclusions and recommendations in relation both to their application to practice and the implications for healthcare. Recommendations in terms of future research agendas are normally included. Other information such as costs involved in treatment regimes should be addressed.

Table 9.1   A selection of systematic review software/tools

Systematic Review (SR) Toolbox	A community-driven catalogue of tools that support the systematic review process: **http://systematicreviewtools.com**
Review Manager 5 (RevMan 5) and the next generation RevMan Web	Software used for preparing and maintaining Cochrane reviews: **https://community.cochrane.org/help/tools-and-software/revman-5**
GRADEPro GDT	Software developed to support the creation of summary of findings tables for systematic reviews, health technology assessments and guidelines: **https://gradepro.org**
EPPI-reviewer 4	Software developed to support all types of literature review, including systematic reviews, meta-analyses, 'narrative' reviews and meta-ethnographies: **https://eppi.ioe.ac.uk**
System for the Unified Management, Assessment and Review of Information (SUMARI)	Produced by the Joanna Briggs Institute, this software is designed to facilitate the entire review process, including protocol development study selection, critical appraisal, data extraction and synthesis: **www.jbisumari.org**
Covidence	Software for importing citations, screening titles and abstracts, undertaking risk of bias assessment and data extraction: **www.covidence.org**

META-ANALYSIS

Meta–analysis is defined by Greenhalgh (2014: 124) as 'a statistical synthesis of the numerical results of several trials that all addressed the same question'. It enables the bringing together of results for studies that are said to be homogeneous in nature – considering the same outcome of the same intervention, on the same population – in an objective way. The effect of combining the results of a number of smaller studies by way of meta–analysis can increase the power of analysis and improve precision and the ability to answer questions not asked by individual studies (Deeks et al., 2011).

Akobeng (2005) proposed that a meta–analysis should have two stages:

1. Calculating a measure of treatment effect (common measures are odds ratios (OR), relative risk (RR) and risk difference – see Table 9.2) and confidence interval for each study.
2. The overall treatment effect is calculated as a weighted average of the individual summary statistics.

The reviewers begin by deciding which of the outcome measures of the studies reviewed are to be used for the meta–analysis – in most studies a number of outcomes are measured,

Table 9.2   Treatment effect measures (Khan et al., 2011)

Measure	Description
Odds ratio (OR)	OR is the ratio of the odds of an event or outcome in the intervention group to the odds of an outcome in the control group.
	An OR of 1 indicates no difference between comparison groups.
	For an undesirable outcome an OR < 1 indicates the intervention is effective in reducing the odds of that outcome.
Relative risk (RR)	Also known as risk ratio. RR is the ratio of the risk in the intervention group to the risk in the control group.
	A RR of 1 indicates no difference between comparison groups.
	For an undesirable outcome, a RR < 1 indicates the intervention is effective in reducing the risk of that outcome.
Risk difference (RD)	Also known as Absolute Risk Reduction (ARR). In comparative studies, it is the difference in event rates between two groups.
Number needed to treat (NNT)	NNT is the number of patients who need to be treated to prevent one undesirable outcome. In an individual study it is the inverse of RD.
Number needed to harm (NNH)	NNH is the number of patients who need to be treated for one additional patient to experience an episode of harm (adverse effect, complication, etc.)

Source: Khan et al, 2011, CRC Press. Reproduced with kind permission of Taylor & Francis.

although only some of these may be of interest to the reviewers. The findings in relation to these outcomes are presented as treatment effect measures, which identify the strength and direction of the relationship between the independent and dependent variables.

The reviewers will also identify what is known as statistical heterogeneity – that is, how diverse the effects are across the various studies. This is usually demonstrated through the use of forest plot graphs – sometimes referred to as 'blobbograms' (see Figure 9.1 for an example).

A forest plot is a graphical representation of a meta-analysis. Each horizontal line represents the results of one study and the square or 'blob' in the middle of each line is the estimated treatment effect of the study (odds ratio, relative risk, etc.). The size of the blob represents the size of the effect, which is usually in proportion to the number of participants in the study; larger studies receive a greater weighting than smaller studies. The width of the line represents the 95 per cent confidence interval of this treatment effect – as identified in Chapter 7, the wider the interval the less precise the estimate. The vertical line is the 'line of no effect' where the intervention group is no better or worse than the control group. In this example, if the confidence interval of a particular study crosses the 'line of no effect' it means that either there is no significant difference between treatment groups and/or the sample is too small to be confident that there is an effect. The heterogeneity of studies can be instantly assessed in forest plot graphs as the more scattered the lines, the more heterogeneous the results. The more heterogeneous the results, the less confidence there is in the ability to use the results in practice.

The diamond below all the horizontal lines represents the pooled effect of combining all the studies. The diamond's position reflects whether overall there is confidence that one treatment is better than the other. On the line means that for the average person there is little choice between the two, while to the left of the line identifies one is better than the other.

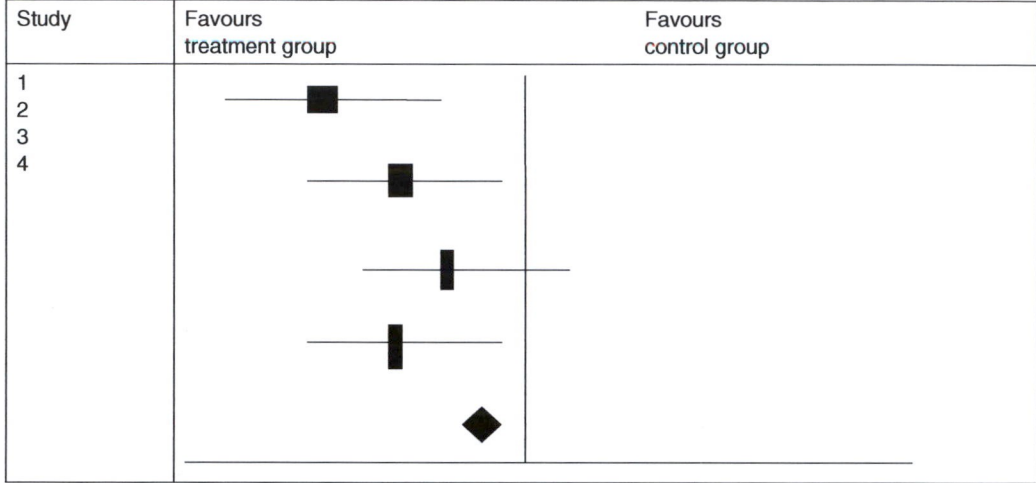

Figure 9.1   Forest plot graphs

If the studies are seen as homogeneous and heterogeneity of treatment effects are identified between studies, Khan et al. (2011: 56) suggest that this may be due to differences in the characteristics of populations, interventions, outcomes or study design. For example, if in one study the sample of older people included those between the ages of 65 and 80 years and in another the sample was made up of those aged over 80, that would represent a heterogeneous population and may explain why differences in the effect of an intervention were seen. Where none of the above is apparent, Khan et al. (2011) suggest that heterogeneity may be a result of publication bias. This type of bias occurs due to a tendency in some areas for only positive results to be published, and when using such findings for systematic reviews a bias towards effectiveness is likely. It is expected that the reviewers should explore this possibility.

It may be the case that individual studies are too small to produce precise effects, but the precision is improved by combining them in a meta-analysis (Khan et al., 2011: 57). The Cochrane logo is a representation of an example of this pooling which identified significance. It represents a meta-analysis of seven RCTs related to the effect of corticosteroids on women expected to give birth prematurely. The first RCT on this subject was published in 1972; however, it wasn't until the publication of a systematic review in 1989 by Crowley that the effectiveness of this treatment was finally recognised. This led to more widespread use of corticosteroids on women at risk of pre-term birth, thus probably saving thousands of premature babies (Cochrane Community, 2017).

> Visit the Cochrane website at www.cochrane.org and view the logo.
>
> **Activity 9.3**

A sensitivity analysis is usually undertaken to identify any changes in the original data that may have occurred as a result of pooling. This involves re-analysing data from different perspectives to see if this has an impact on the results. If substantial changes are reported to have occurred as a result of pooling data, then caution should be taken in applying the results to your own area of practice.

> Visit the Cochrane Library at www.cochranelibrary.com and access a systematic review relevant to your own area of practice and familiarise yourself with the organisation and layout of a systematic review and meta-analysis.
>
> **Activity 9.4**

META-SYNTHESIS

Meta-synthesis is derived from the Greek words *meta* meaning 'denoting change, transformation, permutation, or substitution' and *synthesis* meaning 'a body of things put together; a complex whole made up of a number of parts or elements united' (*Oxford English Dictionary*, 2018). This suggests meta-synthesis is about putting together things in a way that goes beyond the features of the individual items. Finlayson and Dixon (2008) have suggested it is the bringing together of the findings of qualitative research in an effort to provide a clearer picture of the phenomenon of interest. Evans and Pearson (2001) also identified that a meta-synthesis allows systematic and critical examination/ interpretation.

Lachal et al. (2017) suggest that the value of qualitative syntheses is now being recognised in that they allow the 'meanings, experiences and perspectives' of participants to be examined both deeply and broadly. Understanding people's experiences is essential to 'understanding the human experience' and gives patients a voice in the healthcare decision-making process (Joanna Briggs Institute, 2014: 5).

There are a variety of approaches to meta-synthesis; indeed, as Pope et al. (2007) identified, various terms are used to describe the processes (such as interpretive synthesis, meta-study, qualitative meta-analysis). However, Pearson et al. (2007) claim these approaches generally involve:

- data extraction – identifying the research findings in the form of metaphors, themes, categories and/or concepts present within the study;
- data synthesis – grouping the findings into categories;
- grouping the categories into synthesised findings.

The processes involved are very similar to that of primary qualitative research and, as in any form of qualitative research, the reviewers are providing an interpretation of the findings. The process appears on the face of it to be a simple one, but in reality, is quite complex and requires a rigorous examination of the studies. The aim is to provide an accurate representation of the findings, which gives a full picture of the essential characteristics of the phenomenon under consideration. The specific approach used to achieve this is expected to be clearly outlined to enable you to judge the rigour of the process and the appropriateness of the review for application within an area of practice.

Whereas heterogeneity is an issue of great concern within meta-analysis it is less so within meta-synthesis (Evans and Pearson, 2001). In qualitative research heterogeneity is anticipated; the issue for reviewers is to ensure that differences are acknowledged, compared across studies and accounted for within the new interpretation.

Table 9.3   Meta-synthesis approaches (Polit and Beck, 2018)

Approach	Description	Example
Noblit and Hare (1988) (Meta-ethnography)	• Consists of seven phases and focuses on constructing interpretations rather than descriptions. Considers how studies relate to each other (either reciprocal – directly comparable; refutational – in opposition to each other or alternatively in a line of argument) • Translating studies, ensuring main concepts are reflected • Synthesising the various translations into a comprehensible whole • Providing a narrative account of the synthesis	Voldbjerg, S., Grønkjaer, M., Sørenson, E. and Hall, E. (2016) Newly graduated nurses' use of knowledge sources: a meta-ethnography. *Journal of Advanced Nursing*, 72(8) 1751–1765.

Approach	Description	Example
Sandelowski and Barroso (2007)	• Consists of two processes of synthesising qualitative research • Meta-summary is the 'quantitatively oriented aggregation of qualitative research findings that are themselves topical or thematic summaries or surveys of data' (Sandelowski and Barroso, 2007: 17), which can either be the final product or be the initial stage before meta-synthesis • Meta-synthesis is 'an interpretive integration of qualitative findings that are themselves interpretive syntheses of data…' (Sandelowski and Barroso, 2007: 18)	Dam, K. and Hall, E. (2016) Navigating in an unpredictable daily life: a metasynthesis on children's experiences living with a parent with severe mental illness. *Scandinavian Journal of Caring Sciences*, 30(3) 442–457.

However, meta–synthesis is not without its dissenters. There has been debate around whether meta–synthesis of qualitative findings is appropriate or indeed possible. For those that advocate meta–synthesis, some would propose that only findings from studies using the same methodology (phenomenology, ethnography, etc.) are possible, while others would argue that it is possible and appropriate to combine findings from various methodologies. Polit and Beck (2018) identify two approaches to meta–synthesis, which are outlined in Table 9.3.

The generalisability of qualitative meta–syntheses is also debated. As qualitative research itself makes no claims of generalisability, with the emphasis being seen as providing thick description and providing insight into phenomena, there are concerns about making such claims in relation to meta–synthesis of results. Nevertheless, the pulling together of 'like' studies and providing wider consideration of a particular phenomenon in relation to a specific group can have practical uses.

CRITIQUING A SYSTEMATIC REVIEW

Although the process of undertaking systematic reviews is rigorous, this does not mean that they do not need to be critically appraised. As identified in Chapter 6, there are a number of tools available to help you undertake critical appraisal (Appendix 8 provides a generic approach to critically appraising systematic reviews). When critically appraising, it may be helpful to have some research books to hand so that information can be checked or clarified. A number of recommended titles are listed at the end of this chapter.

Activity 9.5

Identify alternative tools/checklists for critically appraising systematic reviews.

Applicability to practice

The criteria identified in Chapter 6 for judging applicability to practice are equally valid for systematic reviews; however, there is also another aspect that should be considered. The specificity of a systematic review question means that a very focused aspect of care is usually being considered and there is a clear need to place this within the context of the care environment in question. Consideration also needs to be given as to whether factors not considered in the review will have implications for applying the results to an area of practice.

Activity 9.6

Identify a systematic review specific to your area of practice and critically appraise it using the checklist in Appendix 8.

Summary

- Systematic reviews provide a rigorous review of research findings in relation to a specific question and as such they are fundamental to EBP, providing nurses and other healthcare professionals with sound evidence on which to base practice.
- The systematic review process involves the 'pooling' of results from 'like' studies and creating a larger data set for analysis. This is known as meta-analysis in relation to quantitative research and meta-synthesis with regard to qualitative research.
- If there is significant heterogeneity within the studies reviewed in a systematic review it is unlikely that the results of the study will be subjected to meta-analysis.
- There are a variety of approaches to meta-synthesis; it is important that a clear description of the approach is provided to allow decisions to be made as to the rigour of the review.

FURTHER READING

Akobeng, A.K. (2005) 'Understanding systematic reviews and meta-analysis', *Archives of Disease in Childhood*, 90(8): 845–8.

Finlayson, K. and Dixon, A. (2008) 'Qualitative meta-synthesis: A guide for the novice', *Nurse Researcher*, 15(2): 59–71.

Gerrish, K. and Lathlean, J. (2015) *The Research Process in Nursing* (7th edn). Oxford: Wiley-Blackwell.

Gough, D., Oliver, S. and Thomas, J. (2017) *An Introduction to Systematic Reviews* (2nd edn). London: Sage.

Khan, K., Kunz, R., Kleijnen, J. and Antes, G. (2011) *Systematic Reviews to Support Evidence-based Medicine: How to Review and Apply Findings of Healthcare Research* (2nd edn). Boca Raton: CRC Press.

Moule, P., Aveyard, H. and Goodman, M. (2017) *Nursing Research: An Introduction* (3rd edn). London: SAGE.

Parahoo, K. (2014) *Nursing Research: Principles, Process and Issues* (3rd edn). Basingstoke: Palgrave Macmillan.

Petticrew, M. and Roberts, H. (2006) *Systematic Reviews in the Social Science: A Practical Guide.* Malden: Blackwell Publishing.

Polit, D.F. and Beck, C.T. (2018) *Essentials of Nursing Research: Appraising Evidence for Nursing Practice* (9th edn). Philadelphia: Wolters Kluwer.

USEFUL WEBLINKS

Campbell Collaboration: an international network that produces systematic reviews and other evidence syntheses in relation to crime and justice, education, international development nutrition and social welfare available via the Campbell Library. www.campbellcollaboration.org

Centre for Reviews and Dissemination: provides guidance on conducting systematic reviews. Also produces PROSPERO, an international register of prospectively registered systematic reviews in health and social care. www.york.ac.uk/inst/crd

Cochrane Library: includes the Cochrane Database of Systematic Reviews, which is the leading resource for systematic reviews in healthcare. www.cochranelibrary.com

EPPI-Centre: undertakes, supports and develops methods for systematic reviews and synthesis of research evidence. Their knowledge library provides a browsable list of systematic reviews in a wide range of fields including education, health promotion and public health. http://eppi.ioe.ac.uk

Joanna Briggs Database of Systematic Reviews and Implementation Reports: a refereed online journal that publishes systematic review protocols and systematic reviews of healthcare research following the JBI methodology. journals.lww.com/jbisrir (subscription required although some article are free).

Conclusion to Part II

The aim of Part II was to provide you with the necessary skills, knowledge and tools to enable you to critically appraise a range of evidence. Hopefully you have now:

- identified a number of papers relevant to your own area of practice;
- found a number of appropriate tools to aid you in your critical appraisal;
- identified gaps in your knowledge and developed action plans to allow you to fill in the gaps;
- developed confidence in your ability to critically appraise evidence in an appropriate way.

Part II ends with a word search puzzle in which there are 21 words associated with Chapters 6, 7, 8 and 9. What are they? The answers can be found on p. 223.

J	T	R	I	A	L	U	O	U	T	Q	T	V	Q	U	X	T	E	V	X
A	G	M	U	Q	V	A	R	I	A	B	L	E	S	E	L	R	O	E	D
S	K	S	Q	Q	L	X	R	I	G	O	U	R	E	B	H	U	M	G	H
K	V	S	J	R	S	J	C	F	D	N	B	T	Y	T	N	S	N	Z	S
K	W	Y	B	F	N	K	O	Q	A	P	F	B	E	R	Z	T	J	R	T
M	A	Z	R	T	O	Q	N	N	Z	R	E	J	U	A	Z	W	D	A	R
O	V	H	A	T	W	E	F	Z	R	O	Z	F	I	N	Y	O	E	N	A
D	S	Y	C	D	B	Y	I	X	E	B	U	F	J	S	H	R	P	D	T
E	M	P	K	W	A	R	R	K	L	A	P	E	Q	F	F	T	E	O	I
R	E	O	E	A	L	E	M	E	I	B	T	T	L	E	F	H	N	M	F
Y	T	T	T	J	L	D	A	F	A	I	K	I	A	R	E	I	D	I	I
A	A	H	I	L	R	V	B	X	B	L	D	C	L	A	W	N	A	S	E
K	A	E	N	D	E	O	I	G	I	I	G	D	N	B	Z	E	B	E	D
E	N	S	G	I	Q	B	L	E	L	T	U	U	L	I	W	S	I	D	S
U	A	I	T	U	R	K	I	E	I	Y	F	G	K	L	Z	S	L	O	S
N	L	S	T	V	P	B	T	Z	T	F	F	Z	U	I	V	E	I	A	B
K	Y	C	W	R	W	J	Y	A	Y	M	E	A	N	T	K	R	T	C	P
L	S	U	J	E	M	I	C	B	A	S	N	K	M	Y	V	W	Y	G	O
S	I	U	F	R	T	Z	Y	P	R	I	V	A	L	I	D	I	T	Y	T
C	S	K	C	R	E	D	I	B	I	L	I	T	Y	T	D	F	R	C	B

PART III
Making Changes

10

Reflection, Portfolios and Evidence-based Practice

Paul Linsley and Janet Barker

Learning Outcomes

By the end of the chapter you will be able to:

- identify the key aspects of lifelong learning;
- apply reflection as an aspect of EBP;
- bring reflective approaches to practice;
- discuss your personal and professional development needs;
- identify key elements of portfolio development

INTRODUCTION

Evidence-based practice is viewed as not only encompassing the use of appropriate research and literature but also embracing lifelong learning, as a way to ensure practice is evidence based. **Lifelong learning** is seen as essential if practitioners are to be able to meet the ever-changing demands of practice (Jivanjee et al., 2015). EBP requires that health professionals' knowledge and skills development keep pace with the demands of practice and evidence development. There is, therefore, a need to develop the skills associated with lifelong learning. **Reflection** and portfolio development are central to this process, as they can enable individuals to identify their learning needs, set goals for that learning and evaluate whether these have been met appropriately. Reflective practice and evidence-based practice are essential to clinical practice. The former provides a retrospective look at current practice and questions the reason for doing so. The latter provides the means by which best evidence can be used to make functionally sound and clinically relevant decisions (Barredo, 2005). This chapter will help you to consider how you can develop the skills of lifelong learning and reflection and ensure your personal and professional development.

LIFELONG LEARNING

Lifelong learning is considered an indicator of what it is to be a professional (Mi and Riley-Doucet, 2016). It provides a framework by which individual professionals can keep up to date with developments in their field, as well as improve their clinical practice and knowledge in line with contemporary thinking. The European Lifelong Learning Initiative defined lifelong learning as:

> … a continuously supportive process which stimulates and empowers individuals to acquire all the knowledge, values, skills and understanding they will require through-out their lifetimes and to apply them with confidence, creativity and enjoyment, in all roles, circumstances, and environments. (Watson, 2003: 3)

Furthermore, it can be considered,

> an attribute involving a set of self-initiated activities and information-seeking skills with sustained motivation to learn and the ability to recognize one's own learning needs. (Hojat et al., 2006)

The above definitions imply a continuous process of learning and engagement, and a willingness to explore new knowledge and understanding as part of everyday practice. It is not something that comes naturally; it takes a personal commitment to pursue learning throughout a professional career (Rishel, 2013). Lifelong learning is about acquiring and updating existing knowledge, skills and qualifications and in turn valuing all forms of learning. Individuals can only develop if they are provided with opportunities to do so and have a predisposition and motivation to explore new ways of knowing. Individuals can only develop as autonomous professionals if they are sufficiently informed, prepared and predisposed to making use of learning opportunities afforded them, as and when they present.

Lifelong learning is more than keeping up to date. Learning to learn and learning about something are two different things. There are two main ways of learning: mediated – aided by a 'teacher' – and unmediated – through experience. Kolb (1984) proposed that learning from experience is a cyclic process whereby experiences are analysed through the use of reflection to promote learning and generate new ways of working. The four stages are experience, reflective observation, making sense of the experience and testing new experiences. It is suggested that the learning process often begins with some kind of concrete experience, professional or personal, that the student considers interesting or problematic. Observations and information are gathered about the experience and then the person reflects upon it, replaying it over again and analysing it until certain insights begin to emerge in the shape of 'theory' about the experience. Boud et al. (1985) proposed that people are often unaware of their learning processes, that reflection made these processes accessible and enabled people to use them more effectively and, therefore, enhance their lifelong learning.

Leaving learning to 'chance experiences' in relation to EBP is not appropriate and a more structured approach, which promotes focused experiential learning through the use of self-direction, is needed. Self-directed approaches come from theories of andragogy (how adults learn) and are implicit within lifelong learning. It is suggested that adults are self-directive in their learning: namely, that they have a readiness for and a motivation to learn, drawing on past experience as a resource for learning. Self-directed learning involves developing the ability to identify what you need to know and how to go about learning it. Knowles (1990) identifies four key factors that should be considered when identifying learning needs:

1. Assessment of needs – reflecting on your experiences to identify where you are, where do you want to be and what is in the gap between the two.
2. Identifying learning goals.
3. Planning how to meet those goals.
4. Evaluating the outcomes.

This, in turn, is based on a number of assumptions about how adults learn (Knowles, 1990: 57); these are as follows:

1. Adult learners bring life experiences to the learning process that should be acknowledged.
2. Adults need to know why they need to learn something, and how it is relevant to their lives and work.
3. Experiential, hands-on learning is effective with adult learners.
4. Adults approach learning as problem-solving.
5. Adults learn best when the topic is of immediate value to their lives.

Evidence-based practice and reflection provide both the foundation and means by which life-long learning is accessed and realised through a cluster of abilities, such as using technologies and finding, using and evaluating evidence, as well as self-analysis and critical thinking. Lifelong learning offers professionals the opportunity to bring up to date their knowledge and understanding of themselves and of their practice. Learning opportunities are all around you in healthcare and it is important to make the most of them. One of the best ways of developing and maintaining a lifelong learning focus is to learn and practise the skills of reflection.

REFLECTIVE PRACTICE

Nurses and other healthcare professionals are encouraged to reflect on their practice and value reflection as part of lifelong learning. This requires them to share good practice with others and engage in continuing professional development through reflection, evaluation and the appropriate use of research. As part of their revalidation process nurses are required to record a minimum of five written reflections on their continuing professional development (NMC, 2017). This process is designed to disentangle the various components of professional practice and allow for personal growth and development through reference to the wider literature and contemporary thinking.

It has been argued that reflection has been going for as long as nurses have cared for patients. It has taken place informally wherever nurses have thought critically about what they are doing and have looked for advice, teaching or support from others. A common-sense view of reflection is that it involves just thinking about things. We each take time out of the day to 'reflect' on what we, and others, did and said; this is only natural and part of human nature. What we do not always do is take it a step further and make plans to do things differently. Purposeful and professional reflection is undertaken with the aim of bringing about a change in either thinking or behaviour.

The concept of reflection can be traced back to the work of Dewey (1933) who described reflection as the 'active, persistent and careful consideration of any belief or supposed form of knowledge in the light of the grounds that support it and the further conclusion to which it tends'. It was popularised by Donald Schön (1990; 1994), who defined reflective practice 'as the ability to reflect on one's actions so as to engage in a process of continuous learning'. Schön studied the ways professionals made decisions and found similarities between people working in fields as different as nursing, architecture and law. In these complex activities, practitioners did not apply rules direct from textbooks. Instead, they linked knowledge from reading with practical knowledge from experience and worked out their own rules for decision making. Schön also noticed that experienced professionals experimented in practice. They tried new ways of doing things, took note of the outcomes and then modified their practice as a result. Schön used the term 'reflective practice' for this process of developing rules for decision making from both academic knowledge and experience, testing them out further through informal academic knowledge and experience, then testing them out again through informal experimentation. Schön's work provides a foundation and introduction to reflection and remains a fundamental component of knowledge and understanding of what it is to reflect.

It is through reflective practice, that learning becomes an experimental approach to individualised challenges that in turn form the basis for further exploration and investigation. This approach is concerned with conceptual change and whether students have reached a certain level of understanding that may be interpreted, for example, as 'thinking like a nurse', and builds on the experiential learning theory's notion of learning by doing, that individuals learn from experience, and that knowledge is valid regardless of the setting in which it took place.

Reflective practice should be viewed as a higher-order thinking skill, such as analysis, synthesis, problem solving, inference and evaluation (King, 1995). Furthermore, 'Reflection is not a normal state of mind' (Bengtsson, 1995: 28), but a disciplined manner of thought that a person adopts to assess the validity of something, and to plan ahead (Miller et al., 1994). It requires constructing knowledge by perceiving a dilemma, exploring the differing perspectives, integrating existing and new knowledge, and considering new alternatives and actions (Patterson and Newman, 1993). It requires insight and self-awareness and a willingness to explore elements of practice and self that the nurse may not be wholly

Table 10.1 Examples of reflective models

Gibbs (1988) reflective cycle	Boud et al. (1985)	John (1995)	Borton (1970)

1. **Description** – what happened
2. **Feelings** – what you thought and felt
3. **Evaluation** – what was good/bad about the experience
4. **Analysis** – making sense of the events
5. **Discussion** – what else could have been done
6. **Action plan** – what to do now
	1. **Experience**
	  a. behaviour
	  b. ideas
	  c. feelings
	
	2. **Reflection**
	  a. consider
	  b. evaluate
	
	3. **Outcomes**
	  a. new perspectives
	  b. changes in behaviour
		1. **Description** of experience – 'what is significant?'
		2. **Feelings** – 'own and others'
		3. **Goals** – 'what was I trying to achieve?'
		4. **Influencing factors** – 'what influenced the way I felt, thought, responded (social, cultural, organisational, cognitive, professional)?'
		5. **Theoretical framework** – 'what theory did or should have informed my actions?'
		6. **Ethical aspects** – 'did I act for the best?'
		7. **Previous experience** – 'how does this link with my previous experiences?'
		8. **Looking forward** – 'how might I do it differently?'
		9. **Framing** – 'what have I learnt?'
			1. **What?** – what is the issue/problem? Asking questions such as what happened, what was I doing?
			2. **So what?** – what does this tell/teach/mean? Asking questions such as 'so what more do I need to know? So what was I thinking/feeling? So what could I have done differently?'
			3. **Now what?** – asking questions such as 'now what do I need to do next time?'

comfortable with. It requires constructing knowledge by perceiving a dilemma, exploring the differing perspectives, integrating existing and new knowledge, and considering
new alternatives (Linsley, 2006). By 'consciously looking and thinking about experiences,
actions, emotions, feelings and responses' we can interpret them so that we can learn, thus
you become more critical about your views of practice and the world (Patterson and
Chapman, 2013). However, reflection is best when pursued with intent and the purpose
of application.

Most nurses are introduced to the concept of clinical reflection as part of their professional training. Nurse education requires students to begin to practise reflectively from the
start of their programme of training. While an integral part of nurse education and clinical
practice, reflection is essentially an individual pursuit. Reflection can be difficult, even
threatening at first, because it forces us to be honest with ourselves and recognise not only
our successes but areas where we need to improve. There are many forms of reflection and
it is individual choice that determines how and what we reflect upon (see Tables 10.1 and
10.2 for examples and different ways of undertaking reflection). While these all share the
same basic elements, the best way to approach reflection is to find a way that suits your
style of thinking and working.

Table 10.2   Different styles of reflection

Method	Types
Individual	Reflective frameworks
	Critical incident analysis
Facilitated	Guided reflection
	Peer reflection
Group	Action learning sets
Clinical supervision	Individual
	Pairs
	Group

Schön (1983) suggested that reflection is undertaken in two ways:

1. Reflecting-in-action – while undertaking activities, during the experience of practice.
   The ability to 'think on one's feet' and apply knowledge and past experience to the
   current situation.
2. Reflecting-on-action – a conscious attempt to reflect after the event.

He also identifies what he calls espoused theory and theory-in-use. Espoused theory is
knowledge that is 'said' to underpin practice and is generally accepted as the appropriate body of formal knowledge on which to base that practice. Theory-in-use represents
the theories *actually* used when practising – the beliefs, values and thoughts that direct
your behaviour. Sometimes the two are very different. For example, if asked about
promoting patient dignity a nurse may advocate the need to ensure privacy, to show

respect for individual wishes and to communicate appropriately with an individual, but in performing a task related to personal hygiene may ignore specific patient preference in relation to religious requirements and so on. Experience is not enough to bring about learning by itself. Nurses and other healthcare professionals need theory that makes sense to them, personally, and which they can relate to practice. This can only be achieved, it is argued here, when nurses share what they have learnt through reflection with others, so that insights, innovations and revelations can be debated, challenged and improved upon. This said,

> External clinical evidence can inform, but can never replace, individual clinical expertise, and it is this expertise that decides whether the external evidence applies to the individual patient at all and, if so, how it should be integrated into the clinical decision. (Sackett et al., 1996: 72)

Reflection can be undertaken in relation to a range of experiences. Often, it will be incidents that are seen as 'significant' – either because something did not go as well as anticipated or because something unexpected happened – that are most likely to prompt consideration. However, it is also important to reflect on the normal, day-to-day events, as these are the ones where practice becomes 'ritualised' and is likely to be based on out-of-date evidence.

Reflection is central to all aspects of EBP, from identifying that there is an issue of concern to implementing changes to practice. Mantzoukas (2007) stated that reflection enables us to unlock the unconscious knowledge on which we base practice, bringing these into our consciousness and thereby allowing our decision-making process to become clear. It also enables us to link the knowledge gained through experience with more formal types of knowledge and to then identify areas of concern. Reflection, as discussed in Chapter 4, is an implicit part of clinical decision making and central to implementing changes to practice.

THE DEEP MODEL OF REFLECTION

Reflective models, as we have seen, can vary in the number of stages they contain and in their complexity (Burnard and Chapman, 1993). Adopting a structured process such as the model below allows the novice to start to reflect on their experiences as well as learn things about themselves. The following model was designed to introduce nursing students to the concept and stages of reflection highlighted as important in the literature. Reflective models are not intended to be used as a rigid set of questions but to act as a prompt for self-questioning and learning.

The idea that reflection is a largely a prediction-making activity underpins the DEEP Model of Reflection. In any course of action, we generate predictions and explanations about ourselves and others' behaviours and how we might respond to them in different contexts. In this way, reflection allows the nurse to consciously consider their experiences and employ new ways of knowing in their clinical practice. It should also be remembered that reflection is not an end in itself but a starting point on which to build and develop.

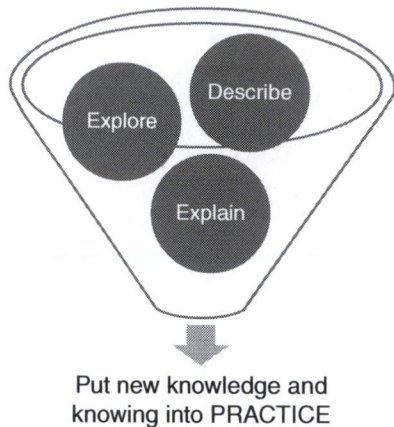

Put new knowledge and
knowing into PRACTICE

Figure 10.1   The DEEP Model of Reflection

Description (What actually happened?)

As with most models of reflection the DEEP model asks the student to provide a descriptive account of the thing they are reflecting on. This means returning to the experience and providing a detailed recounting of the event. This helps clarify the student's thinking and bring to the surface easily assessible attributes. It is important at this stage to identify exactly what the key elements are, in other words, *what makes this an incident worthy of reflection?*

Exploration (What was its impact on you?)

The learner starts to ask questions and to connect ideas together as to why things happened the way they did by exploring the situation in more depth. This includes attending to feelings, both positive and negative, and exploring why they might have felt that way. Exploration can be a painful experience, bringing things to consciousness that need dealing with. The memory of a challenging situation includes an affective component, which at times may be difficult to handle. Some incidents may be so challenging that they create a great deal of uncontrolled emotion and cathartic support may be necessary before an attempt to think positively or constructively becomes possible. It is through this process that the student not only explores elements of their clinical practice but facets about themselves.

Explanation (What did you learn from the experience?)

Knowledge, or knowing, is created through the preceding two steps by nurses consciously considering their experiences and providing an account of their actions and thinking. This third step requires the practitioner to explain their actions and beliefs, thoughts and feelings with reference to the wider literature and others. It is through this process that the practitioner can get to know themselves in terms of (1) easily accessible surface attributes, (2) less directly accessible attributes such as beliefs, and (3) reasons for their behaviours and beliefs. Knowledge creation requires curiosity and a willingness to ask questions of oneself. It also needs the practitioner to be honest about doubts and uncertainty or lack of knowledge. Reflection goes beyond just gaining knowledge and challenges us to explore the foundations on which our knowledge is built. It also allows us to strengthen our understanding of a given situation or practice as well as increase our self-awareness of the values and attitudes that influence our knowledge and how we use this to inform what we do and why we do something. As we become capable of generating more and more plausible explanations for our thoughts and actions, we achieve more self-identities and possess more self-knowledge. As Jenny Moon (1999) suggested, reflection is used 'with the sense of saying something not so much about what a person does as what they are about'.

Put into Practice (What did you decide to do as a consequence of what you learnt?)

The last stage of most models of reflection relates to a willingness to change practice, where new conceptual perspectives are reached in order to inform practice. Reflection builds upon experience deliberately, allowing us to interpret and incorporate new ideas through the integration of theory with practice, and in turn with praxis, through experience (Barker and Linsley, 2016). These new ideas if not rejected by practitioners become working principles; the implications of which are further tested through experience and subsequent modification after further reflection. If we are not willing to change practice we will not gain the potential benefits from the process in terms of practice development, advances will not be made, and professional practice will not evolve. By following the process, reflection allows the practitioner to explore their strengths and examine personal development needs, while at the same time allowing them to plan ahead and engage in new and modified experiences (Clarke et al., 1996). Reflection starts with the individual or group and their own experiences and can result, if applied to practice, in improvement of the clinical skills performed by the individual through new knowledge gained on reflection. Reflection can lead to constructive action in relation to planning, implementation and evaluation of change (Page and Meerabeau, 2000). However, there needs to be a clear link between reflection and actions – making changes to one's own behaviour will not come about without a clear and proactive action plan and the motivation to put the plan into action.

In reflection there is no 'one size fits all' approach and as identified earlier you need to consider what works well for you. There are, however, a few basic things that need to be put in place to be successful:

- Experiment with different approaches until you find one that 'fits'.
- Commit to giving time to reflection in whatever form you choose – see it as an essential aspect of your practice rather than an 'add on'.
- Start small and work up to the big issues.
- Be open to new ideas and new ways of thinking.
- Be willing to challenge your assumptions and practices.

REFLECTIVE WRITING/JOURNALS

Reflection can be done by thinking through things in a structured way; however, writing reflectively can add another dimension to the process. There is something about taking thoughts and reproducing them on paper that provides greater clarity and insight into an experience and leads to a deeper learning experience. It supplies a way of ordering your thoughts and freely expressing your feelings and concerns. It also helps to structure your experience and to make links between various ideas and concepts. You can consider issues in a more objective way, returning to the account of your practice at a later date if necessary without having to rely on being able to fully recall all the details. If you reflect regularly in a reflective diary, for instance, it can provide a log of your activities and allow you to consider if there are recurrent issues that need to be considered in more depth.

Reflective writing should be a creative process that allows full expression of thoughts and feelings, enabling you to explore and clarify the issues surrounding your experience. Therefore, it is expected that you write in the first person – 'I did…' – so that you 'own' the experience. One of the barriers to reflective writing is that often writing is seen as part of a specific process (education programmes, practice reports, nursing notes) and, therefore, people learn to write in a way that is required by others (teachers, mentors, managers). However, this reflective of writing is aimed at meeting your needs and you should find a way of doing this that you feel comfortable with. As with all reflection it needs to be structured if it is to aid in your learning, and so you need to find a model that will help you to do this. Like all other skills you need to practise this regularly to feel confident in doing it; don't worry that you 'might get it wrong', rather concentrate on finding a way that feels 'right' for you. It is useful to identify specific times when you will reflect and if you are able to make it part of your routine this will soon become an essential component of your practice. It may also be useful, when in the practice setting, to have a pocket notebook with you so you can jot down thoughts and issues as they happen, so you can reflect on them later. It is important to remember that reflective accounts are a private record of experiences, and so it is important to capture your thoughts, feelings and opinions as well as merely the factual events that took place. And that,

> The personal–practical knowledge acquired through reflective learning that mediates healthcare delivery and that cannot be pinned down completely in protocols and procedures needs to be captured and developed. (Hyde, 2009: 119)

A reflective journal is a way of capturing your thoughts and feelings in a critical and analytical way. Reflective journals allow you to review your development over time and can help in identifying gaps in your knowledge and skills and in thinking about how you might go about addressing these. They also provide evidence of learning and a means of promoting oneself. As with reflection, a journal is a personal matter and should be organised to suit the individual and their learning needs.

CLINICAL SUPERVISION

Reflection can be undertaken on an individual basis or as part of clinical supervision. Clinical supervision first appeared in nursing some 30 years ago, being proposed as a way of helping nurses to cope with the demands of healthcare delivery. It gained momentum as it became seen as a way of facilitating aspects of government initiatives in relation to clinical governance and encouraging continuing professional development and improvement through a formal process of professional support. It has also been endorsed by the NMC as a way to improve standards of care and is intended to be a career-long undertaking. The Department of Health (1993) defined supervision as:

> A formal process for professional support and learning which enables individual practitioners to develop knowledge and competence, assume responsibility for their own practice and enhance consumer protection and safety in complex situations. It is central to the process of learning and scope of the expansion of practice and should be seen as a means of encouraging self-assessment, analytical and reflective skill.

Furthermore, it is 'a process of professional support and learning that enables practitioners to develop knowledge and competence to improve care' (McColgan and Rice, 2012: 36). As such, clinical supervision provides a safe environment in which the practitioner can discuss their practice and their personal and professional development and is aligned to life-long learning principles. Clinical supervision is undertaken between two or more people, with one person identified as the clinical supervisor, and involves reflection-on-action and the implications of this for future care delivery. Usually, the clinical supervisor will have undergone some form of training to prepare for their role. The aim of the supervision is to discuss and explore an aspect of practice or a particular issue in depth in an attempt to understand what has happened and if different approaches are feasible/possible/available. The clinical supervisor challenges the supervisee's ways of thinking and working, while at the same time providing a safe and supportive environment. There are various models available; however, the most commonly used are:

1. Educative (formative approaches) – aimed at developing a better understanding of individuals' skills, action and the patient experience.
2. Supportive (restorative approaches) – considers emotional responses and the experience of delivering care.
3. Managerial (normative approaches) – explores quality issues and ensures appropriate standards of care.

All the approaches usually involve the agreeing of a contract that stipulates the format, length and timing of meetings, confidentiality and the recording of discussions. Many NHS trusts have policies in place identifying their expectation of staff in relation to clinical supervision and the form it will take.

PORTFOLIO

Portfolios have been around for a number of years and have been particularly embraced by nurse education. Various definitions are available. McMullan et al. (2003: 289), for example, defined portfolios as 'a collection of evidence, usually in written form, of both the products and processes of learning. It attests to achievements and personal and professional development, by providing critical analysis of its contents'. The aim is to create an organised and ordered document that illustrates the person's professional skills and strengths and more importantly, personal growth.

As McMullan et al. (2003) identified, they are usually in written form; however, electronic portfolios are becoming increasingly popular.

There are four main reasons for producing a portfolio:

1. Learning and development – to demonstrate progress over time.
2. Professional development – to meet statutory requirements to demonstrate you have kept up to date (e.g. for the NMC).
3. Assessment – as part of a course to enable an assessment of learning.
4. Presentation – to showcase your achievements, for example at an interview.

Portfolios are seen as a way of actively engaging people in their own learning, providing a vehicle through which to explore the process and provide evidence of learning.

Portfolios also promote self-directed learning and development, requiring you as a learner to take control of, and responsibility for, your own learning. In turn, they provide a framework for reflecting on your personal and professional development. Most nurses will have had experience of keeping a portfolio as part of their formal education – if you are a pre-registration student or a newly qualified nurse you will no doubt have been required to keep one in some shape or form. The advent of the Agenda for Change career structure (DH, 2006b) and the identification of the Knowledge Skills Framework both indicated that a portfolio of some kind is needed to demonstrate learning and the meeting of agreed developmental goals for registered nurses. Using this to direct your own learning in relation to EBP can seem a daunting task. However, there are key approaches that can be adopted to direct your activities – a possible framework is proposed below:

1. Reflect on a practice issue to provide a view of where you are and where you want to be and, therefore, your learning needs.
2. Identify learning goals to be achieved through the use of frameworks such as SMART
3. Undertake a SWOT analysis to help you to identify which issues are likely to impact on your ability to meet your goals (see template in Appendix 1); this will enable you to generate an action plan (see template in Appendix 9) to achieve your goals.
4. Implement the action plan, collecting 'evidence' of your learning.
5. Evaluate your progress and adapt your plan as you develop.
6. On meeting your goal(s) the process can begin again.

If the above steps are followed and the documentation is completed it will provide you with a portfolio of your development and learning over time and enable you to both monitor and provide evidence of your progress.

PERSONAL DEVELOPMENT PLANNING

Personal development planning is viewed as a structured approach by which individuals can reflect on their current knowledge, skills and achievements, and plan their personal and professional development needs. Mulhall and Le May (2001) propose that to make the transition to EBP there is a need for individual nurses to actively plan their own personal and professional development to ensure that they have and maintain the necessary skills and knowledge associated with their area of practice. This includes thinking about your developmental needs in terms of further study and experience. A template for a personal development plan is provided in Appendix 10 and it may be worth considering what your education and training needs are to ensure you have the skills and knowledge to be an effective practitioner capable of EBP.

Summary

- Lifelong learning, reflection and portfolio development are central aspects of EBP.
- People are often unaware of their learning processes; reflection makes these processes accessible and enables people to use them more effectively.
- Self-directed learning involves identifying what you need to know and how to go about learning it.
- Reflective practice has three elements – experience, reflection and action – and thus provides a structure through which to consider experiences.
- There are three approaches to clinical supervision – educative, supportive and managerial.
- Portfolios provide a framework through which to structure learning.
- Personal development planning is a structured approach to reflect on current knowledge, skills and achievement, and plan personal and professional development needs.

FURTHER READING

Bolton, G. and Delderfield, R. (2018) *Reflective Practice: Writing and Professional Development* (5th edn). London: Sage. This book provides an excellent recourse, particularly when capturing your thoughts as part of reflective writing.

McKinnon, J. (2017) *Reflection for Nursing Life: Principles, Process and Practice*. London and New York: Routledge. This book provides a good overview as to the importance of reflective practice and offers practical models and frameworks to support reflective practice.

USEFUL WEBLINKS

The Royal College of Nursing: Eight ways to improve your reflection. www.rcn.org.uk/professional-development/revalidation/eight-ways-to-improve-your-reflection

11

Evidence into Practice: Practice Development, Improvement and Innovation

Paul Linsley

Learning Outcomes

By the end of the chapter you will be able to:

- define the terms improvement and innovation;
- discuss the key features of practice development;
- discuss the need for practice innovation;
- identify how to introduce new evidence into the practice setting;
- discuss various approaches and challenges associated with the management of change;
- consider how to develop an evidenced-based culture in the practice setting.

INTRODUCTION

The last 20 to 30 years have seen a proliferation of changes in the way that healthcare services are delivered and structured. This has been in response to a number of factors. Changing demographics, greater economic freedom, an increase in life expectancy, advancements in treatments and technology, changing patterns of migration, changes to family structures and changes to the way we work, have all meant a rethink in the way in which we access and deliver health and social care. In order to meet these changes there has been a growing emphasis on defining standards of practice, implementing evidence-based practice and pursuing innovation and improvement in organisations and clinical teams. In this way, healthcare services are seldom static but operate in a state of flux – they respond to changes in public demand and are sensitive to the politics of the day.

Practice development, improvement and innovation are seen as an integral part of today's healthcare system and the answer to modern-day demands. Perhaps the biggest challenge faced by staff today is the need to provide a high standard of care within increasingly limited budgets. Judicial use of the available evidence and research is of great importance when supporting claims of practice improvement and innovation. It is apparent that EBP has become firmly established in guiding practice-based decisions and interventions and that it represents a key approach for developing and sustaining high quality, patient-centred care. However, achieving quality, improvement and efficiency is a complex activity that requires careful thought and attention. These issues will now be explored and the importance of EBP highlighted when responding to changes in practice.

> Before reading the rest of the chapter, consider what the terms improvement and innovation mean to you. Can you give examples of each based on what you have read in the literature or observed in clinical practice?
>
> **Activity 11.1**

PRACTICE DEVELOPMENT

A wider choice of different types of health services is increasingly becoming available to patients to enable personalised care, faster treatments and personal support through the processes of practice development. A number of definitions have been used to describe practice development; perhaps the best known of these is that put forward by Kitson (1994: 319) who described it as:

> a system whereby identified or appointed change agents work with staff to help them introduce a new activity or practice. The findings may come from the findings of rigorous research; findings of less rigorous research; experience which has not been tested systematically or trying out an idea in practice. The introduction of the development ought to be systematic and carefully evaluated to ensure that the new practice has achieved the improvement intended.

Furthermore, it is:

> a continuous process of developing person-centred cultures. It is enabled by facilitators who authentically engage with individuals and teams to blend personal qualities and creative imagination with practice skills and practice wisdom. The learning that

occurs brings about transformations of individual and team practices. This is sustained by embedding both processes and outcomes in corporate strategy. (Manley et al., 2008: 9)

In this way, practice development plays a pivotal role in fostering a culture and context that nurtures evidence-based practice because it is an:

> approach that synthesises activities and theory of quality improvement, evidence-base and innovations in practice, within a real-practice context, and with a central focus on the improvement of care and services for patients and clients. (Page and Hammer, 2002: 6)

Over time the term practice development has become associated with supporting the modernisation of healthcare and covers a wide range of activities designed to move practice forward in a timely and orderly manner. Practice development can be said to have the following key characteristics (Caldwell, 2004: 215):

- It incorporates a range of approaches.
- It takes place in real practice settings.
- It is underpinned by the development and active engagement of practitioners.
- It is collaborative and interprofessional.
- It is evolutionary.
- It is transferable rather than generalisable.
- It focuses on the improvement of patient care.

Practice development covers such activity as quality improvement, practice innovation, the setting and monitoring of standards, and staff development and training. In this way, practice development draws on and synthesises theory and activity from a number of fields and disciplines, such as evidence-based practice, clinical audit, satisfaction surveys, emergent research, and national guidelines issued by professional and government bodies.

PRACTICE IMPROVEMENT

While the two terms, innovation and improvement, are often spoken about together, there needs to be an understanding as to their uniqueness. Improvement is any action that seeks to change things for the better while innovation is the introduction of a new way of thinking or working. An improvement could be made in the way patient care is administered, the way in which a service is delivered, or individual performance and knowledge. Practice improvement has been defined as:

> The combined and unceasing efforts of everyone – healthcare professionals, patients and their families, researchers, payers, planners and educators – to make changes that will lead to better patient outcomes (health), better system performance (care) and better professional development. (Batalden and Davidoff, 2007: 2)

In order to develop practice there is a requirement to not only consider what we are doing, but why we are doing it. The model for improvement (Institute for Healthcare Improvement, 2015) asks three questions:

1. What are you trying to achieve?
2. How will you know a change is an improvement?
3. What changes can you make that will result in the improvement that you seek?

Practice improvement can involve examining the way in which a service is run, the way in which staff practise, as well as the way in which patients are treated. The goal of practice improvement is to achieve a higher quality experience for patients (Maher and Panny, 2005). Improvement thinking involves four equally important and interrelated parts that are essential for improvement activities, these being:

- personal and organisational development: building a culture that supports improvement;
- process and systems thinking: understanding work processes and systems, and the linkages within them;
- involving users, carers, staff and the public: understanding their experiences and needs;
- making it a habit: initiating, sustaining and spreading, building improvement into daily work. (Penny, 2003)

Achieving improvements in clinical practice requires the collaborative effort of the team and all members should feel empowered to contribute. However, this is not always easy to achieve. Healthcare services are seldom static – they evolve over time as the attitudes of those that use the service change with developments in thinking and technology. Some changes are not intentional while others are desired and required. Increasingly, changes are being made quickly and do not allow for a period of adjustment, which can leave staff feeling powerless and not engaged with. It is important to remember that: 'Not every change is an improvement but certainly every improvement is a change and we cannot improve something unless we change it' (Goldratt, 1990: 10).

The utilisation of evidence is a core element of EBP, although this is not without its difficulties. The transferring of evidence into practice is often a daunting, difficult and complex activity. Simply informing people of the latest research findings does not automatically result in new approaches being adopted and it cannot be assumed that developments in knowledge and skills will result in changes to practice. For instance, most people know that hand washing is central to reducing infections and yet large numbers of health professionals fail to do this appropriately (see, for example, Haas and Larson, 2008). Changing care delivery and individuals' behaviours and approaches takes time and effort. It is important to be thoroughly prepared before trying to instigate changes. There is no single best way of introducing new evidence into practice, as the type of change required will often dictate the approach to be used.

In order to facilitate change there needs to be an understanding as to the complexities of health and social care and recognition that neither is static but evolving. Central to this whole process is the patient. It is, therefore, important that any intervention or improvement should be based on the needs of those that use the service. There is a need to work flexibly and across different groups and to look at the reasons that have tended to underline poor practice, these being:

- inconsistent standards – between practitioners, departments and organisations;
- barriers between services
- inflexible, unresponsive services
- over-centralisation and the disempowerment of patients and staff (Page, 2002)

When thinking about change we are encouraged to focus on the three areas below:

1. *Structures* refer to the geography and lay out of facilities and equipment, organisational boundaries, roles and responsibilities, teams, committees and working groups, targets and goals.
2. *Processes* refer to patient journeys, care pathways, educational processes, funding flows, recruitment of staff, procurement and supporting processes such as ordering, delivery and dispensing.
3. *Patterns* refer to patterns of thinking and behaviours, conversations, relationships, communication and learning, decision-making, conflict and power. (NHS Institute for Innovation and Improvement, 2005)

Before any change can be initiated a plan is required that identifies the reason why the change is needed and how it will be carried out. There are a number of improvement frameworks and models to guide the clinician in practice. All make use of data to evaluate needs and opportunities, refine solutions and monitor outcomes. A popular model is the Model of Effective Implementation. This follows a straightforward and systematic process whereby information and data are collected in support of the proposed change, the change is planned for and then introduced, following which it is evaluated. Grol et al. (2013) offered the following model for effective implementation:

1. Research findings/guidelines (the evidence is gathered)
2. Matching problems identified or best practices (current practice is evaluated against 'best practice')
3. Describing specific change targets
4. Analysis of target group, current practice and context
5. Development/selection of strategies (a plan is put in place)
6. Development and execution of implementation plan
7. Continuous evaluation and adapting plan

Any improvement in a service tends to be spoken of in terms of quality. Quality is complex and contains a number of elements and means different things to different people. The Institute of Medicine stated that,

> quality of care is the degree to which health services for individuals and populations increase the likelihood of desired health outcomes and are consistent with current professional knowledge. (Institute of Medicine, 2001)

What is often referred to as the six dimensions of quality highlights that healthcare should be safe, effective, patient–centred, timely, efficient and equitable (Institute of Medicine, 2001). These six dimensions continue to inform and act as a benchmark when developing services not only in the UK but also across the world.

> Look at an improvement in your area of interest. What drove this improvement? How did it come about? What evidence underpinned its introduction? How was its impact measured? Did it achieve all its aims?
>
> **Activity 11.2**

PRACTICE INNOVATION

Innovation comes from the Latin roots of the word, 'in–nova–tion' which literally means 'in a new way'. Nurses are in an ideal position to change and challenge practice as they provide most of the care delivered worldwide. Innovation involves thinking about new ways of doing things. It requires us to think creatively and flexibly to generate new ideas to solve old problems. Innovation is when a creative idea is put into action and has been defined as:

> The intentional introduction and application within a role, group, or organisation, of ideas, processes, products or procedures, new to the relevant unit of adoption, designed to significantly benefit the individual, group or wider society. (West, 1990)

This definition captures the three most important characteristics of innovation: (a) novelty, (b) an application component and (c) an intended benefit (Lansisalmi et al., 2006). It implies a real change in the way that things are done and a desire to move practice forward. It requires a commitment to improvement and service development and should be based on sound and demonstrable evidence. Healthcare innovation can be defined as:

> ... the introduction of a new concept, idea, service, process, or product aimed at improving treatment, diagnosis, education, outreach, prevention and research, and with the long-term goals of improving quality, safety, outcomes, efficiency and costs. (Omachonu and Einspruch, 2010)

For the purposes of this book, we prefer a much simpler definition of innovation, and define it as:

> An idea, service or product, which significantly improves the quality of health and care wherever it is applied. (DH, 2011: 9)

The intended benefit from a patient's perspective is either improved health or a reduction in suffering due to illness (Faulkner and Kent, 2001). Innovation comes in many forms. There are innovations in the way systems are organised and managed, technological advancements and new treatments and interventions. Innovation is not just about having a good idea, however. It is about putting this idea into practice. This requires the development of the idea, successful deployment and the sharing of this work with others. There are three important stages to getting an idea into practice, these being:

- *Invention* – The originating idea for a new service or product, or a new way of providing a service
- *Adoption* – Putting the new idea, product or service into practice, including prototyping, piloting, testing and evaluating its safety and effectiveness
- *Diffusion* – The systematic uptake of the idea, service or product into widespread use across the whole service. (DH, 2011)

Once effective healthcare innovations are identified, effective approaches to disseminate these practices need to be developed. This includes guidelines for the use of effective health practice, disseminating this information, and providing technical assistance to aid health organisations and practitioners changing established practices and adopting new innovations.

Innovation has to be more than a simple improvement in performance – it needs to be radical in the way it sets about tackling a problem or be a real advancement in the way that we think or do something. Conversely, there is an important role for what is termed 'reverse innovation' – this is the decommissioning of an activity that is shown to have no added value or that has been replaced by something new or better. There are different types of innovation, and they do not always need to be 'big ideas'.

- Product – changes in products or services
- Process – changes in the ways products or solutions are created and delivered
- Position – changes in the context in which products or solutions are introduced
- Paradigm – changes in the way that we think about things.

Each innovation type can occur at different levels:

- Incremental – small step changes, occurring on a day-to-day level
- Modular – significant changes in one element, within an overall architecture that remains unchanged
- Discontinuous – a change in the established methods
- Architectural – the introduction of new frameworks of operation. (Tidd and Bessant 2017)

Activity 11.3

Visit the Gov.UK Research and Innovation in Health and Social Care site at the following address: www.gov.uk/government/policies/research-and-innovation-in-health-and-social-care.

Look at the sort of things that are highlighted as being innovative practice. A lot of the innovations are centred on the use of information technology and advances in treatments and medicines. Think about your own practice. What do you consider to be innovative? It may be something as simple as a new way of working

WHAT DOES MOVING FROM EVIDENCE INTO PRACTICE MEAN?

EBP is an essential element to moving practice forward and an important component in service development, innovation and improvement. While EBP is generally accepted as something to aspire to, in reality changes to practices are not easily made. Understanding the complexities of change and, in particular, achieving sustainable change is useful when thinking about getting evidence into practice. Timmins et al. (2012) found that a number of issues impacted on nurses' use of research findings in practice. These relate to a lack of time to engage in EBP activities such as finding relevant up to date research; limited skills in relation to application of research to practice; and a perceived lack of support from colleagues and managers coupled with an apparent reluctance to adopt new practices by some. The time between evidence being generated and practice being adopted in a setting could be significant. Often practices will be considered safe, having been based on evidence, but frequently this will be out-of-date theory.

The reasons why valid evidence and clinical guidelines are not routinely adopted into practice are often complex and involve both the individual and organisation. Rycroft-Malone et al. (2004b) identified four main reasons to explain why this reluctance might exist, they are:

1. Inability to interpret research findings.
2. Lack of organisational support.
3. Research seen as lacking clinical credibility.
4. Nurses preferring a clinical specialist to tell them of the latest developments.

Thompson et al. (2008) argued that nurses preferred to rely on experiential sources of knowledge. Yadav and Fealy (2012) support the idea that nurses rely on this experiential knowledge and clinical expertise gained through their own and others' experiences. This type of knowledge is valued because it is specific to the context in which nurses work, as well as readily accessible and patient-centred. Research, on the other hand, tends to be seen as less easy to access, and often not specifically relevant to the sorts of issues nurses are faced with. Nurses also appear to prefer others (such as nurse specialists) to provide them with research evidence rather than seek it out themselves.

Consider one area in which you have had clinical experience. Identify those factors which would help and those which would act as barriers to making changes in practice.

Activity 11.4

Straus and McAlister (2000) suggest that implementation of evidence–based change requires the development of new skills. Moving people out of their 'comfort zone' is not an easy task and can be at the heart of whether change is successful or not. Concerns may relate to beliefs (either real or imagined) about what the change will mean for them and come from:

- fear of the unknown;
- uncertainty about the value of the change;
- a lack of knowledge and/or skills;
- a lack of confidence in ability to meet new demands;
- feelings of powerlessness;
- resentment if change is seen as unnecessary.

Activity 11.5

Imagine that you have been told you need to change a particular aspect of your practice. What feelings would this evoke and what would be your most likely response?

Moving evidence to practice involves a number of complex interactions (Wilkinson et al. 2011), not all proposed changes occur and there are a number of barriers to successful implementation of changes:

- Perception of research/evidence – this has to be seen as legitimate.
- Staff factors – lack of experience, knowledge, skills.
- Organisational issues – structure, management systems.
- Resources – equipment, staff and so on are not available.
- Patient/carer perceptions – preference, level of knowledge, availability of information.

Five 'pearls of wisdom' are offered by Butz (2007), which give a starting point for developing EBP and implementing changes into practice at a personal and team level as well as creating an EBP culture:

1. Personal development – making a commitment to accessing databases on a regular basis.
2. Team discussions – timetabling regular meetings with colleagues to discuss ideas, information and to identify areas for change.
3. Culture of enquiry – promoting and developing an enquiry approach in your area of practice.

4. Research relationships – encouraging the development of relationships that may result in research activities.
5. Disseminate evidence – creating systems for sharing information and best practice evidence.

> Consider the five 'pearls' above. Chose two and identify how you could build these into your work life.
>
> **Activity 11.6**

It is clear that any attempt to change should be planned for and actively managed. Any proposed change needs to involve all those who will be affected by it and this, in turn, will inform the circumstances in which the evidence is disseminated and introduced into the practice setting. Dissemination activities by themselves are unlikely to lead to changes in behaviour; however, this should not be taken to mean that raising awareness of the messages underpinning proposed changes is unimportant. Implementation has its own specific areas for consideration. Metz et al. (2007) suggest that there are three types of implementation:

1. Paper – where policies are in place but no changes to practice actually occur.
2. Fragmented – new structures are put in place but not targeted at the right people; therefore, those involved are unable to develop the necessary skills and again practice remains unchanged.
3. Impact implementation – where strategies and structures are appropriate and are designed specifically to ensure practice change.

In implementing change there is a need to ensure that all these have been taken into consideration and addressed before attempting to make a change. There is also a need to check progress frequently and ensure feedback is given to people at regular intervals, so they are aware of progress and any issues that have arisen. If changes to practice are to be sustained and the practices implemented remain in place, there is a further need to ensure that the necessary resources are maintained, and people are rewarded for doing a good job.

The PARIHS (Promoting Action on Research Implementation in Health Services) framework developed by an RCN project group (Rycroft-Malone, 2004) draws together three elements that are thought to be central to the success of making changes to practice:

1. Evidence – its clarity.
2. Context – its quality.
3. Facilitation – type needed.

For change to be successfully brought about, the evidence on which changes are to be based needs to be high quality, valued and viewed as relevant by both the clinical staff and patients/service users. Grol and Grimshaw (2003) noted the characteristics of the evidence can have a major influence on whether it is integrated into practice, and that some forms of evidence are easier to integrate into practice than others. If evidence reflects widespread concerns in relation to particular practices, or is seen as supporting professional group values, then it is more likely to be adopted. The quality of evidence also impacts on uptake, for example guidelines that are clear, explicit and straightforward are more likely to be implemented.

Once a body of evidence on a particular issue which has implications for practice has been identified, there is a need to evaluate and synthesise this evidence to identify what needs to be done in relation to the specific area of interest (Fineout–Overholt et al., 2010c). Once the relevant evidence has been critically appraised (see Chapter 6) and a summary sheet of the relevant papers created (see Appendix 5) this will give an indication of the key aspects of the evidence and which papers are or are not applicable to practice. The implications of integrating these findings into practice and whether or not this has broader implications for others will need to be considered. Any proposed changes will require careful planning and should be discussed with colleagues to ensure the identification of any potential difficulties with the process of implementation.

The context in which care is delivered is itself constantly changing. Patients come and go, their conditions change or may deteriorate rapidly, and working with other healthcare professionals brings its own complexities. If change is to be made against this sort of background there is a need for individuals to feel valued, for necessary resources to be readily available and for effective teamwork practices to be in place.

In implementing change there is a need to ensure that all these factors have been taken into consideration and addressed before attempting to make a change. There is also a need to check progress frequently and ensure feedback is given to people at regular intervals so they are aware of progress and any issues that have arisen. If changes to practice are to be sustained and the practices implemented to remain in place, there is a further need to ensure that the necessary resources are maintained, and people are rewarded for doing a good job.

If change in practice is to happen then it needs to be facilitated by someone. The type of facilitation and the facilitator her/himself are central to the process, which needs to be enabling and empowering and must include all the involved parties in the decision-making process. Change at a team level and beyond therefore needs to be facilitated by someone who is prepared to take on the role of a **change agent** supported by senior members of staff.

Rycroft–Malone's (2002) work suggested this needed to be someone who is part of the team and present in the day-to-day activities, who can see the change as appropriate and can, therefore, motivate individuals. The characteristics of a good facilitator can be seen in Box 11.1.

Box 11.1   Characteristics associated with a good facilitator

- Flexibility
- Persistence
- Negotiating skills
- Facilitation

- Credibility
- Leadership
- Good communicator
- Commitment
- Presence
- Project management
- Persuasive
- Sincerity
- Clarity of vision

It is proposed that the knowledge/skills associated with the change agent role are developed slowly, in a step-by-step and often haphazard way (Greenhalgh, 2014). So, when participating in facilitating changes to practice it is important to start in a small way and develop the skills and approaches over time.

The process of implementing evidence-based practices

Table 11.1 Models for promoting change

Brady and Lewin (2007)	Lewin (1951)	Metz et al. (2007)
1. **Plan** – involve all affected by the change. Identify outcomes. Pilot proposals. Identify motivators.	1. **Unfreeze** – recognition of need for change.	1. **Exploration** – change/ implementation ideas considered.
2. **Implement** – establish a realistic time line with built-in evaluation points.	2. **Moving** – making the change by altering behaviours or activities.	2. **Preparation** – resources needed identified and made available.
3. **Correct** – be flexible and address issues as they arise.	3. **Refreeze** – embedding the changes in practice.	3. **Early implementation** – initial adjustments to implement practices made.
4. **Communicate** – use multiple ways of keeping people informed.		4. **Full implementation** – all staff have appropriate level of competency and change is fully embedded in activities.
5. **Evaluate** – identify impact of changes for both professionals and service users.		5. **Sustainability** – skills, knowledge and resources are maintained at required level to ensure changes remain in place.
		6. **Innovation** – consideration of adaptations and other changes required.

There are various models available to guide the process of changing practice (see Table 11.1 for examples). They all have certain aspects in common, including the need for planning, implementation and evaluation strategies to be in place.

Table 11.2   PDSA Cycle

Stage	
Plan	What are the objectives?
	Who will do what, when, where and how?
	How will you evaluate progress/what data will you collect?
Do	Implement plan
	Note any problems/issues that arise throughout the implementation
Study	Analyse data collected
	Compare data with objectives
	Identify what you have learnt
Act	What do you want to achieve next?
	How will you

An approach commonly used with NHS service improvement initiatives is the PDSA cycle (Plan, Do, Study, Act). This is based on the work of Deming (1986) and reflects the scientific process of hypothesis (Plan), experiment (Do) and evaluate (Study). See Table 11.2 for an overview of this. You might also consider that this is also like a nursing approach to patient care: hypothesis (plan) [assess need], experiment (do) [implement care], evaluate (study) [reassess/evaluate care], act [continue to implement care which delivers positive outcomes for the individual].

Iles and Sutherland (2001) suggest that it is important that these aspects are not seen as being separate and discrete stages that are undertaken in isolation. It is likely, no matter how thorough the planning, that issues will arise which have not been considered; therefore, planning must remain a continuous process. The implementation phase needs to be evaluated at all points to ensure that what is intended to happen, does indeed do so.

As issues arise, further planning and then implementation will be needed, with an evaluation of the impact of adjustments made. As Schön (1994) describes, there are areas of professional practice where evidence can be easily used to support practice – the high hard ground; however, more frequently practice occurs in 'messy' and 'swampy lowlands' where there are challenging problems which will frequently impact on the rigorous application of evidence to practice.

The planning stage usually involves what is known as a diagnostic analysis. As Nickols (2016) suggests, change is a problem-solving activity, which usually starts with a diagnosis of the problem, allowing goals to be identified and strategies by which these can be achieved put in place. The 'problem' considered in relation to EBP is the moving from one practice to another and, therefore, the diagnostic analysis will involve a consideration of the area or context within which change is to be made. The idea is to identify any barriers and organisational and/or professional issues which must be taken into account before any attempt is made to implement change. This also allows for the identification of the gap between what is currently happening and what the vision for the future is. Highlighting the gap makes planning the implementation easier and also reduces the likelihood of unforeseen problems and barriers to changing practices arising.

One of the simplest and easiest approaches to consider the issues around making a change is to use a SWOT analysis – Strengths, Weaknesses, Opportunities and Threats. An alternative to SWOT is the 7S model presented in Table 11.3.

Table 11.3   7S Model

Element	Features
Staff	What is needed – number, skill mix, characteristics (attitudes, values, etc.)?
Skills	What is needed and what are available in relation to: • clinical/technical skills? • interpersonal skills? • managerial skills? • research/EBP skills?
Structure	What are the current features of the organisation? What is needed? What is the 'fit' between the two?
Systems	What is in place and what is needed?
Strategy	What is the plan? What are the priorities?
Style (management)	What is the current style? Does this fit with what is needed to achieve the planned changes?
Shared beliefs	What beliefs and values are present? What is needed to achieve the planned change? Is there a gap between the two?

Identify an area of practice that you would like to change and use either a SWOT (a template is provided in Appendix 1) or 7S model to identify the issues you would need to consider.

Activity 11.7

An alternative to these two models is the 'how, what and why' approach. These question types reflect the various approaches to change that different people take within organisations – namely their 'mindset'. Working through these questions can help to address all the issues that need to be considered and planned for.

- How do I get colleagues to change from X to Y intervention?
- What do I want to achieve, what changes have to be made, what will indicate success?
- Why is X intervention used and why do we need to change to Y?

Activity 11.8

Consider the SWOT or 7S analysis you undertook in relation to your chosen area of practice. Does the 'how, what, why' approach provide information you hadn't considered?

Once all the issues that may impact on implementing change and the resources needed have been identified, planning how to make the change is undertaken. There is a need here to set realistic goals, to identify a time line and draw up an implementation strategy. Changing practices takes time, and all those that the change will affect should be involved, with time to ensure there is adequate consultation and planning.

McLean (2011) contends there is also a need to manage the psychological impact of making the transition from one practice to another. As transitions involve 'endings' it is necessary to consider how best to manage these. She suggested a five-step model, which acknowledges the psychological impact implicit in moving from one practice to another. Often, people experience anxiety and worry about the implications of changes, and without a clear vision of why practices are 'ending' may view previous ways of working through 'rose tinted glasses'. There are three phases to transition: 'ending', when 'old' practices are stopping; neutral, where 'old' practices have not completely finished and 'new' practices are not fully embedded; and a 'beginning' phase when the new practice is fully implemented. McLean (2011) asserted that a transition facilitator and/or team should be set up to ensure the transition runs smoothly.

Once the change has been fully integrated into practice there is a need to formally evaluate the implementation of the practice, identifying whether the change has had an appropriate impact on care, the lessons learnt and whether further innovations are needed. It is crucial to know whether or not the intended point has actually been arrived at and whether the planned change is an improvement on previous practices. Evaluation needs to be planned as part of the process of introducing new practices and taking decisions in the planning phase as to what is intended to be evaluated – the effectiveness of the practice, the processes used, the impact of the changes, or all three.

Practice development and improvement uses research and theory in a way that is sensitive to practice issues on the ground. Practice development methodologies address:

- facilitated approaches to improving practice;
- development of leadership attributes and skills;
- development of team effectiveness and new ways of working;
- evaluation of changes in workplace culture and the context of practice delivery.

Methodologies include, for example, action research, evaluation research, investigative inquiry, practice inquiry, integrative inquiry and evidence-based practice. Perhaps the most often used of these is evaluation research. Evaluation is recognised as a research approach in its own right and is used extensively in both health and education to maintain and improve the quality of programmes. In its broadest sense, evaluation is a systematic process to understand what a programme does and how well the programme does it (Weiss, 1998). Furthermore, it is the examination of events or conditions that have (or are presumed to have) occurred at an earlier time or that are unfolding as the evaluation takes place. In order to do this, these events or conditions must exist, must be describable, and must have occurred or be occurring. Evaluation, then, is retrospective in that the emphasis is on what has been or is being observed, not what is likely to happen (Rossi et al., 2004: 10).

Evaluation is said to be 'useful' when it provides feedback that can be understood and used by a variety of audiences, including staff, managers, client-groups and other interested parties (Rossi et al., 2004). While assessing the outcomes of a service or intervention is important, outcomes mean different things to different people. If a service has specified goals or objectives, then an obvious outcome is to assess whether these have been achieved. A serious shortcoming of this tight objectives-linked approach is that services and interventions involving people are notorious for having unanticipated consequences (either in addition to, or instead of, the proposed ones). Increasingly, researchers and staff are using different approaches to evaluation; while many of these maintain an element of outcome evaluation, they seek to evaluate other elements of the programme or intervention.

It is clear that any attempt to change should be based on evidence, use a systematic approach and involve planning, active monitoring and evaluation. Any proposed change – for example, a change of practice based on new research – would involve the development of an appropriate dissemination and implementation strategy, clearly articulating the need for change and the strength of evidence on which it is based. This should include plans to monitor and evaluate the degree to which the proposed change has been achieved and its effects, together with methods to maintain and reinforce any change, including the removal of barriers to change. Greater insight is needed into the personal skills and attributes of those being asked to make the change as well as those being asked to lead the change. It may be useful to consider sharing the experience of making changes with a wider audience, writing up the project for publication or presenting it at a conference. A wider dissemination through publication/conference presentation may help others struggling with similar problems, while at the same time adding to the evidence base for nursing practice.

Summary

- In order to move practice forward there needs to be a commitment to innovation and improvement and the development of practice.
- Service development helps to identify best practice by focusing on continuous improvement.
- Both innovation and improvement imply doing; change is an active process.
- The transferring of evidence into practice is a complex activity, which takes time and effort.
- Comfort zones develop over time and change is unlikely unless nurses are motivated to change established practices.
- A shared vision is needed if change is to be successful and people need to have the skills and to see the benefits of implementing a new practice.
- Change can occur on a personal, team, organisation, national or even global level.
- Strategies and structures need to be designed specifically to ensure practice changes are sustained.

FURTHER READING

NHS England (2017) *Building a Knowledge Enabled NHS for the Future*. London: NHS England.

USEFUL WEBLINKS

The Health Foundation: this organisation has a specific interest in the implementation of evidence into health and social care practice. Take time to explore their site: www.health.org.uk

The Point of Care Foundation: this charitable organisation works to provide the tools and support for individuals and organisations to bring about change in clinical practice. www.point ofcarefoundation.org.uk

12

Clinical Academic Careers

Christine Jackson and Ros Kane

Learning Outcomes

By the end of the chapter, you will be able to:

- briefly describe the historical context around the move to degree-level education in nursing, midwifery and allied health;
- define what is meant by the term clinical academic;
- identify potential routes to becoming a clinical academic;
- discuss the contribution that clinical academic staff can make to evidence-based practice.

INTRODUCTION

The engagement of healthcare staff in research has been shown to be associated with improved healthcare performance (Boaz et al., 2015). Indeed, the ability of healthcare professionals to engage in critical inquiry and implement research findings is imperative, and there are many examples of where this makes a significant difference to care experience and clinical effectiveness (HEE, 2015). Clinical academic careers provide a relatively new way of achieving this as well as supporting the nursing, midwifery and allied healthcare workforce in the delivery of evidence- and values-based practice. Clinical academics maintain their practice role while also carrying out research, placing them in a unique position to make connections between research and clinical practice, and to pose new research questions arising from their clinical observations and experience. Professionals who develop a clinical academic career can play a significant role in cultural and behavioural change within organisations and are hallmarked by their leadership potential around the area of evidence-based practice. Training paths for clinical academic roles have existed across the UK since 2006 and clinical research is a fast-growing career pathway for many healthcare workers. However, aspiring clinical academics still face a range of challenges in balancing the clinical and research aspects of their careers, and in applying for and succeeding in opportunities afforded to them. Many clinical academic staff must carve out their own career pathways and influence their workplaces to enable and support their dual practice/ research role, so developing as autonomous practitioners. Influencing and leadership skills are key, as well as developing excellent research skills applied to the particular contexts in which they are working.

As with the expansion of the nurse's role (see Chapter 1) the introduction of evidence-based practice challenged the way in which clinicians are educated and supported. In 2006, a key document from the Department of Health in England set priority areas for modernisation, which included updating career pathways and choices (DH, 2006a). This modernisation programme recognised that healthcare was changing and so too was the healthcare workforce. By the mid-2000s, nursing had become an all-degree profession across the UK. One of the key outcomes from the transition to degree-level qualification was the need to refocus academic research and clinical practice through the creation of opportunities for an innovative career pathway that combined a strong clinical focus together with the benefits of research training. Evidence-based practice was promoted as a means of facilitating this change and fed directly into the development of specialist practitioner roles; for example, non-medical prescribing, practice education and teaching. The role of the clinical academic can be seen as a further development in response to these changes in practice and education. With the generation, interpretation and implementation of evidence being key concerns, clinical academics are well placed to contribute to the improvement of practice, but in order for nurses and other health professionals to engage in research activity, they need to have access to appropriate education and training. Lifelong learning and continuing professional development are important concepts and have a central part in developing a competent and flexible workforce. Nurses and other healthcare professionals need to be made aware of the real opportunities contained within the clinical academic role and how to access them.

This chapter examines the historical development of the clinical academic role and outlines examples of current practice. Presented below is a description of the historical context and subsequent policies leading to the development of the current clinical academic career pathways in England for nurses, midwives and allied health professionals. Allied health professions refer to those professions located within the statutory framework of the Health and Care Professions Council (HCPC). There are currently (2018) 16 health and care professions sitting within the HCPC (see: www.hcpc-uk.co.uk/aboutregistration/ professions/ for a full list and additional information about the role of each profession).

WHO ARE CLINICAL ACADEMICS?

It is important to define what is meant by a clinical academic within nursing, midwifery and allied healthcare professions. The definition used here was formulated by the National

Institute for Health Research (NIHR) and adopted by the Association of UK University Hospitals (AUKUH) for use with their online resource, *Transforming Healthcare* (2016), which provides a focal point and guide when thinking about the implementation and development of clinical academics, and is as follows:

> Clinical academics are clinically active health researchers. They work in health and social care as clinicians to improve, maintain, or recover health while in parallel researching new ways of delivering better outcomes for the patients they treat and care for. Clinical academics also work in higher education institutions (HEIs) while providing clinical expertise to health and social care. Because they remain clinically active, their research is grounded in the day to day issues of their patients and service. This dual role also allows the clinical academic to combine their clinical and research career rather than having to choose between the two.

Activity 12.1

Before reading any further, take time out to identify a clinical academic who might be working in your area. 'Interview' them and reflect on their role; is it a career that might interest you?

The case study below details the experience of a senior academic who previously worked clinically as a therapeutic radiographer. The experience is very typical of clinicians with an interest in developing their research skills, prior to the introduction of the concept of a clinical academic career and the availability of training opportunities.

Case Study 12.1

'I always enjoyed my clinical work and the rapport one develops with patients. The drive you have, to help and support patients through a rewarding career in healthcare, never leaves you but at the same time I wanted something more. That is why I moved from clinical practice into academia. For a number of years, I enjoyed the very different challenges that academia brought and almost 30 years after qualifying, I gained my PhD. Looking back on what I, my colleagues, and peers considered a successful career, my one regret was that I lost my clinical focus and my clinical skills. I missed the patients too. If I were qualifying today, I would hope to take a different career pathway. I would have applied for a clinical academic position and would have undertaken a clinically based PhD study much earlier in my career. This would have allowed me to retain a clinical focus with patients and in addition act as a role model for future aspiring clinical academics. Perhaps, I would go on to either lead a research group or become a consultant practitioner.'

Senior academic, therapeutic radiographer

AN HISTORICAL PERSPECTIVE

Historical perspectives on the development of education and training for nurses, midwives and allied health professionals

Nursing as a profession has been recognised for over 150 years, with the first training school established in 1860, the Nightingale Training School for Nurses at St. Thomas' Hospital in London. One of the first institutions to teach nursing and midwifery as formal professions, it was dedicated to communicating the philosophy and practice of its founder and patron, Florence Nightingale. Nursing qualifications later moved from certificated to diploma training and the majority of training schools were under the control of Health Authorities (the then government agency that was responsible for NHS care in a particular area), with the academic staff in the schools of nursing remaining as NHS employees. A similar approach was taken by those professions considered under the umbrella of allied health, including radiographers, physiotherapists and occupational therapists. Training schools for allied health professions were becoming established throughout the latter part of the twentieth century and were largely single discipline, geographically attached to the larger hospitals, with academic staff drawn from clinical practice who, as with nursing and midwifery, remained as NHS employees (though notable exceptions were the Universities of Edinburgh and Salford where degree programmes in radiography were offered as early as the 1960s).

This structure afforded very clear and direct opportunities for the clinical departments, clinical staff and training schools to work effectively as a unit supporting the students. This close working partnership ensured the availability of opportunities for staff in the training schools to retain their clinical skills and knowledge. Clinical and training heads of service were mutually supportive and often served on hospital management committees together. This encouraged a two-way flow of expertise and information, which in turn benefited the students. However, students – particularly in nursing and midwifery – were considered part of the workforce rather than being supernumerary and this was beginning to cause concern for the professional and registration bodies in place at this time.

Criticisms of the NHS training school structure began to emerge in the 1980s and were wide-ranging. Concerns were expressed by the then Department of Health and Social Services and professional bodies that undertaking diploma-level qualifications through a single-discipline training programme was becoming an outdated approach to training students across healthcare. Considerable discussion took place about the lack of research utilisation in clinical practice and the need to change traditional working practices in keeping with contemporary thinking and a changing health and economic landscape.

The majority of training schools had no links with higher education institutions and were not in a position to benefit from wider academic expertise or multi-disciplinary education at Bachelor level through to Masters and PhD qualifications. During the 1980s, staff in training schools, where the majority held diploma-level and higher professional qualifications, began seeking additional academic qualifications via university programmes. This exposure to the higher education system and the graduate community was providing, for many training staff, an insight into and experience of a wider, formalised academic environment where the principles of learning centred on education rather than training.

In nursing, students were not supernumerary to the clinical nursing workforce, which meant they were often considered as an unqualified member of staff and learnt much of their practice from direct clinical experience. The move to higher education and to degree-level nurse education was arguably an attempt to develop a culture of research awareness, and to provide support and guidance in the development of research skills and the application of research in clinical practice. It also allowed nursing to be placed on a similar footing to other professions (such as physiotherapy), which had embraced degree-based education much earlier. Similar moves are being seen today with paramedic and operating department practitioner training now also being taught at degree-level.

MOVING TOWARDS GRADUATE PROFESSIONS: POLICY INITIATIVES (1980-2000)

Nursing and midwifery

In the 1980s and 1990s pre-registration courses were criticised for their failure to adequately equip students with the necessary knowledge and skills to assume the role of a qualified nurse (Maben and Macleod-Clark, 1998; Bradshaw and Merriman, 2008; Glen, 2009). This provided impetus for the radical reorganisation of nurse education in the UK and the introduction of a new nursing curriculum (Jasper, 1996). The two decades between 1980 to 2000 saw a defined shift in focus for education and training programmes in nursing and midwifery. In 1986, the United Kingdom Central Council for Nursing, Midwifery and Health Visiting (UKCC) (the then professional governing body in the UK), launched Project 2000, which aimed to move nursing education into the higher education sector and create a single tier of registered general nurses (RGN) in contrast to the previous two-tier registration: the State Enrolled Nurse (SEN), which required a two-year training programme, and the State Registered Nurse (SRN), which a required a three-year diploma programme of study. It proposed to educate a 'knowledgeable doer' capable of both giving and supervising nursing care. The aim was to produce a mature and confident practitioner who was able to accept responsibility, think analytically and flexibly, be able to recognise a need for further preparation, and was willing to engage in self-development (UKCC, 1986). Project 2000 became the driver for the transfer of schools of nursing and midwifery into higher education institutes and set a route to enable the diploma qualification to be phased out and replaced by pre-registration undergraduate programmes in nursing and midwifery. Nurse training, therefore, moved away from the traditional 'apprentice-style' education to a diploma-level curriculum built upon firm theoretical knowledge (Glen, 2009).

In the late 1990s, Project 2000 came under scrutiny as experienced health professionals expressed concerns about levels of fitness to practise among newly qualified nurses (Maben and Macleod-Clark, 1998; Gerrish, 2000; Higgins et al., 2010). These concerns led to an examination of the Project 2000 curriculum and the formation of two documents named *Making a Difference* (DH, 1999) (which also applied to midwifery education) and *Fitness for Practice* (UKCC, 1999), and also the publication of recommendations to strengthen pre- and post-registration education and training in the UK (Higgins et al., 2010). *Making a Difference* (DH, 1999) and *Fitness for Practice* (UKCC, 1999) provided the foundation for new curricula and the move towards all-degree education (Higgins et al., 2010).

Allied Health Professions

Although there were some early successes in terms of developing pre-registration degree programmes (the first undergraduate programme in Physiotherapy was validated at the University of Ulster in 1976), the majority of the other allied health professions had to wait considerably longer for success (Price, 2009).

During the late 1970s, the Boards of the Council for Professions Supplementary to Medicine (CPSM), now known as the Health and Care Professions Council (HCPC), together with representatives across education and health from the four UK countries, set up the Higher and Further Education Working Party to consider pertinent issues in healthcare education and training. In 1979, the working party published *The Next Decade* (1979), which made 60 recommendations. One of these was the transfer of funding from the health sector to education, which would bring allied health professions in line with the funding mechanisms in medicine and dentistry. This report might be considered as the impetus for the professional bodies to begin reviewing existing pre-registration qualifications with a view to moving towards a graduate entry for allied health professions. However, it took several more years of debate and discussions with stakeholders across health and education before the professions began to see progress towards approvals for undergraduate pre-registration programmes.

The publication of *Working for Patients* (DH, 1989) through Working Paper 10, on the future of education and training, outlined the case for radical reforms of the organisation of NHS training schools with a view to transferring the management and funding mechanisms to the education sector. This working paper provided the impetus for all allied health professions in existence at this time, along with their professional bodies and the CPSM, to work with then national degree awarding body, the Council for National Academic Awards (CNAA) to validate and accredit pre-registration undergraduate programmes.

> **Activity 12.2**
>
> Take time out to search the history of your profession and how it has developed. What is expected from the professional of the future? How much expectation is there that research should be integral to clinical activity? How much preparation and assistance are offered to support the development of research skills and expertise?

DEVELOPING RESEARCH SKILLS

History and policy context for Clinical Academic Careers

The previous section provided a brief overview of the reforms to pre-registration education and training programmes for nurses, midwives and allied health professionals, detailing the move from the health sector into the higher education system in the UK. Education within the university environment brings recognised benefits. Undergraduate students are now exposed to a multi-disciplinary environment and are part of a wider cohort of university student body with a national voice. The students have access to world-class educational technology to support their learning and are within a research-rich environment. Healthcare academics within schools of nursing, midwifery and allied health are drawn largely from the professions. Healthcare education must retain a strong professional focus and be able to measure professional competence, and students must be confirmed as fit to practise at qualification. The students benefit from research-informed teaching and are afforded opportunities to engage in research prior to qualification.

Moving to an all-degree profession was arguably one of the key actions in modernising nursing. It not only raised the standing of the profession but the expectations of its workforce, including the ability to engage in and implement the findings of research, and this has been reflected in a number of national reports. Recent reviews of educational provision have re-ignited the debate about the content of programmes, with specific reference to the coverage of research topics. For example, in England, The Shape of Caring review (2012), commissioned by Health Education England in partnership with the Nursing and Midwifery Council, published recommendations for the future education and training of nurses. The final report from the Shape of Caring review, *Raising the Bar* (2015), argued that more needed to be expected from future graduate nurses and recommended that greater acquisition of skills, previously considered advanced or post-registration, should be included in pre-registration programmes. This included the routine application of research and innovation. The review also called for more nurse-led research to ensure evidence-based practice becomes more embedded, which in turn will improve quality of care. To do this, nurses need the knowledge and analytical skills to make informed decisions and contribute effectively to new innovations, taking a more proactive role in service improvement change and change management. The importance of research at pre-registration level is also acknowledged in the new NMC outcomes (2018b), which reflect the proficiencies for accountable professional practice that must be applied across the standards of proficiency for registered nurses, which explicitly state that newly qualified nurses must 'demonstrate an understanding of research methods, ethics and governance in order to critically analyse, safely use, share and apply research findings to promote and inform best nursing practice'.

As a result of the above policy drivers, undergraduate nursing programmes are now required to provide education in research and students are expected to be consumers of research on qualifying.

There are calls for increasing numbers of nurses to undertake Masters and Doctoral level study, and exposure to research experience during undergraduate training as well as the utilisation of research in clinical practice can only support this ambition. Indeed, increasing numbers of registered nurses are engaging with research and, more importantly, seeking to implement research findings to underpin daily work (Shape of Caring review, 2015). However, this is not seen as the norm and applies particularly to early-career nurses.

Increasingly, nurses and other healthcare professionals are taking on extended roles (previously the remit of the medical profession) requiring changes in their skill set and knowledge. Nurses need to acquire a strong grounding to develop a questioning approach to care that encourages them to question inappropriate care practice and to adopt an adaptive and innovative approach to care that seeks to impact positively on patient care experience. There are opportunities for academic staff to gain higher-level clinical and academic qualifications and indeed this is now a requirement for all healthcare academics. Although nursing, midwifery and allied health professional (NMAHP) research is relatively underdeveloped, and the 'clinical academic' workforce is estimated at only 0.1 per cent of the NMAHP workforce in the UK (AUKUH, 2017), the number of doctorally qualified healthcare staff is increasing and the health sector is working towards a target of 8,500 by 2020 (AUKUH, 2017).

While the benefits of undergraduate education are recognised for both students and academic staff, it is important to discuss concerns around the transition from hospital-based schools to the higher education sector.

The transition to degree-level qualification from diploma necessitated, for most training establishments, a geographical relocation into a local higher education institution (HEI). The relocation of the schools to HEIs places an additional burden on both clinicians and academic staff in terms of distance and, therefore, travelling times to meetings and supporting students in practice. Geographical isolation affects the ease with which healthcare professionals across the sectors interact and, therefore, maintain effective communication. In addition to this, many clinicians were concerned that provision of a graduate education would impact negatively on the clinical aspects of training and there was a concern that graduating students would be less clinically competent than their diplomate predecessors. These concerns were recognised by academic healthcare staff and there are systems in place to address these concerns. All undergraduate healthcare programmes are required to ensure that graduating students undertake a minimum number of hours of supervised and assessed clinical practice. Students are required to pass the clinical component prior to admission to the requisite professional register. There is a strong drive for theoretical components of programmes, including research modules, to be grounded in clinical practice. In order to better support this, clinicians are asked to support students by giving clinically relevant lectures, with some clinicians being offered honorary contracts with HEIs. Many HEIs now have clinical skills laboratories where students gain valuable clinical training skills relevant to their specific profession.

Healthcare academic staff who were part of the reforms seen in the 1980s and 1990s had to make adjustments to their professional development when the transfer to HEIs took place. The new profile for academic healthcare staff brings new tensions relating to their diverse responsibilities and accountabilities. They have had to gain academic qualifications (Bachelor degree through to PhD) to add to their professional curriculum vitae, integrate into a very different educational environment and support students undertaking new programmes. In addition to this, there are pressures on all academic staff to undertake and publish research in order to be recognised in the Research Exercise Framework (the formal system for assessing the quality of research in UK higher education institutions).

This period of transition for the academic healthcare workforce was for some academic staff an opportunity to develop their wider ambitions and move into leadership positions outside of their professional area. During the 1990s new professorial positions were created, and appointments of deans of faculties and heads of college drawn from within the healthcare professions. Despite these notable leadership appointments, there was no coherent strategy to support career pathways development for healthcare academics recently repositioned into HEIs. At the same time, the schools of nursing, midwifery and allied professions received assistance from colleagues from NHS organisations in terms of offering specialist clinical teaching sessions and collaborative leadership support. Healthcare professionals from HEIs and the NHS could see that working effectively together by sharing expertise could bring mutual benefits to both communities and undergraduate students.

Local initiatives were developed across the four UK countries, with joint appointments created between trusts and HEIs and there was an emerging interest from clinical staff to undertake academic qualifications to support their continuing professional development. However, these achievements and collaborative arrangements were taking place without any direct and targeted support at a national level. Experienced clinicians attracted to a part-time role within a local HEI, found that differing pay scales and pension providers were barriers to developing a clinical academic career. HEIs were not able to match the salaries paid to experienced clinicians. There were problems with attempting to put together, for example, an honorary contract to allow clinicians to work in the education sector. Difficulties of co-ordinating activity across the health and educational sectors are still visible today and, more recently, recommendations have been made around defined working arrangements, with specific reference to developing and sustaining clinical academic careers. These are discussed further below.

> **Activity 12.3**
>
> Read the case studies below from two health professionals embarking on their clinical academic careers. Reflect on the relative benefits for both health and educational organisations.

> **Case Study 12.2**
>
> 'In a clinical academic career, I think you can have the best of both worlds. You can be in practice but also have the research skills to either drive research and evidence-based practice in your area, or be part of it.'
>
> Nurse, Pre-PhD training programme participant

> **Case Study 12.3**
>
> 'I don't see myself as a clinical academic yet: I'm on the process of starting that journey. That's where I want to end up, but I am not quite there yet. ... I have learnt about my own qualities that I didn't know were there. It has made
>
> *(Continued)*

(Continued)

me feel up to date in my current area of practice by just having a chance to read and reflect. I'm more confident in my everyday interactions, taking on different things and approaching things with less doubt. I know that I have got involved with more research in my clinical area ... I have been involved in national research groups and attended more research events. This has made me more aware of what research is happening in the trust. I am more interested in reading around what is going on and bringing things that I find interesting to team meetings. I hear what's going on in the wider world of things: the courses I can go on, what's happening both nationally and in my local area. It has given me a new passion for what I am doing. Due to this, I had the confidence and motivation to set up my own journal group; we now have that culture where we are looking at new ideas and challenging what is going on. There has never been anyone to carry that through but now I've taken on that challenge and have the confidence to give it a go and see what comes from it.'

Nurse, Pre-PhD training programme participant

EARLY DEVELOPMENT OF INFRASTRUCTURE FOR CLINICAL ACADEMIC CAREERS

In 2003, the Department of Health and the Department for Education and Skills, through its joint Strategic Learning and Research Advisory Group, commissioned a Project team led by Professor Tony Butterworth, then the Chief Executive of the Trent Workforce Confederation, to develop an HR Plan to support educators and researchers across health and social care in the UK. National stakeholder consultations were undertaken and, in 2004, a Strategic Report (StLaR Plan Phase II Strategic Report) was published. The report made 15 recommendations, which are summarised collectively below:

- Develop flexible clinical academic employment models with pre-approved employment contracts together with transparent and accessible guidance relating to employment rights and pension transfer across the 'public sector pensions club'.
- Adopt key proposals from the Follett Review (2001), for medicine and dentistry where an individual retains a single key employer with joint appraisal and job planning mechanisms.
- Support consultant and advanced practitioners to fulfil their full obligations towards education and research, and support managers to work with their employees to consider flexible career options in education and research.
- For clinical trainees in medicine and dentistry, create a specific training pathway, which recognises the academic component through the National Training Number (NTN) Academic scheme.
- Improve the labour market intelligence system to provide accurate data on the disposition of the research and educator workforce for health and social care.

This report was presented to and received by the joint Strategic Learning and Research Advisory Group in 2004. It was agreed that further work should take place in order to build and expand on its recommendations.

In 2005, Sir Mark Walport was commissioned by the Department of Health to make recommendations for the future training of researchers and educators in medicine. This included creating a range of clinical academic training programmes in medicine. The report was written within the context of the UK but it was acknowledged that each of the four countries may wish to adapt the recommendations.

In nursing, the UK Clinical Research Collaboration (UKCRC) tasked Professor Tony Butterworth and Dr Christine Jackson (authors of the StLaR Plan Phase II Strategic Report) to develop the StLaR HR Plan further with a series of recommendations. This resulted in the publication of the 'Finch' Report (UKCRC, 2007), which was later adopted by the Modernising Nursing Careers initiative and was supported by the Chief Nursing Officers across the four countries within the UK. Although the title of the report reflects an initial remit to develop recommendations for the nursing profession, it was always the intention of the authors to include midwifery and allied health professions within the funding processes supporting these recommendations. The central and underlying principle of the recommendations was a vision for a flexible career pathway which places at its core a continued clinical career which is supported through targeted research training from Masters-level degree programmes, such as the Masters in Clinical Research, through to pre-professorial specialist research training.

The recommendations addressed three main areas: **education and training, facilitating careers** and **better information**. In relation to **education and training**, a progressive pathway was recommended to support clinical academic staff to progress though the various levels of a clinical academic career. Awards were recommended at different levels with, for example, first-level awards intended to support early career healthcare professionals wishing to develop their clinical research skills through a defined research masters programme, right through to higher-level awards intended to support post-doctoral clinical academics and prepare them for professorial and leadership positions.

In relation to **facilitating careers**, recommendations were made around supporting career flexibility to encourage rather than hinder careers which bridge both health and education sectors. They were based around the development of a model contract of employment for clinicians to take up research and academic roles without detrimental effects to salary and pension status and to find creative solutions, such as the use of honorary contracts in addition to substantive contracts with clearly defined and agreed roles, timeframes and appraisal systems. The report also acknowledged the importance of good mentorship in the support of aspiring clinical academics and those in more senior positions too. In medicine, there is a long-established tradition of appointing mentors to recipients of the equivalent awards in medicine. The Academy of Medical Sciences (AMS) supports all awardees in medicine through the management of the mentoring processes. The mentoring scheme is regarded as one of the crucial factors in the success of the training programmes, and establishing an equivalent mentoring scheme for healthcare professions was considered to be vital for the success of clinical academic training initiatives.

With regard to better information on nurse researchers, the recommendations for this section of the report related to promoting clinical academic careers to students on undergraduate programmes, healthcare managers and policy makers at local and regional levels.

Activity 12.4

Read the case studies below, which are extracts from interviews with health professionals who had recently embarked on a pre-Masters or a pre-PhD level clinical academic training programme. Reflect on the extent to which exposure to the training has already started to impact on the outlook and confidence levels of these clinicians and how evidence for changing practice is emerging.

Case Study 12.4

'Being on the clinical academic pathway has made me recognise the skills I have got and the potential for those skills. There are a lot of really exciting opportunities to do something different and really make an impact. It [the training] gives you time out of the clinical workspace to consider where you want to go. I think it makes you more critical about what you do in practice, and why all the questioning and enquiring and being critical changes you as a person. My outlook is different now. I think it's about identifying what the issues are and being able to do something about them. I've been able to suggest to my managers ... "let's do a project". In previous years, I might not have had the skills or the confidence to say, "I've got these skills and I can use them ... let me put a project plan together, show you what the potential is". I can now recognise the value of these skills and highlight how they should be valued by the organisation in which I work. Whenever you learn something new, that changes your practice'.

Nurse, Pre-Masters Programme participant

Case Study 12.5

'A clinical academic career gives you the opportunity to contribute academically to your clinical role. I was looking for a different direction and the role was re-animating and re-energising. It has given me the opportunity to stand back and take a broader perspective of my clinical and professional life; and the direction I wanted it to go in. The role has increased my confidence in decision making but also my sense of achievement and motivation to achieve. I am now more inclined to take part in research as a clinician because I realise how difficult it is to get people to contribute to your research. I realise there is a lot out there still to learn, and that has elevated me a little bit and piqued my interest more. My confidence in being able to judge other people's assertions, with regard to research and new ideas, has increased considerably; and now I don't take things on face value quite so much, I mostly check things for myself.'

Paramedic, Pre-PhD Programme participant

'A clinical academic career is about being clinically aware of research and being able to access information that could inform practice and help to move practice on. I think you have to be responsible for yourself in your practice. If you say as a nurse that you are evidence based in your practice, then you have to have some time to actually explore that. I didn't initially see myself as an academic as I hadn't really done much research. I wouldn't have attended research forums or conferences as I wouldn't have thought it was for me. Now I will go and I will expect to come away with something that will help my practice or that I can pass on.'

Nurse, Pre-Masters Programme participant

'The role has given me more confidence to feel like I could make a difference, to want to make changes and to want to influence practice, but also, to make my own judgements. I wouldn't have had the confidence to be as challenging if I hadn't gone through the process of having two papers published; doing the research, being confident in my practice and in how I was delivering things. I think it's also about the confidence and the knowledge of where to go with what I don't know. I've built a network of people that I can tap into, my behaviour of resourcing and sharing has made an impact on how my clinical team perform. There are national guidelines and tools that some of the people in the team didn't even know about. I am now able to share that knowledge.'

Nurse, Pre-Masters Programme participant

CURRENT PROVISION

The reports described above brought clinical academic careers onto the political agenda and paved the way for tangible developments and the beginning of opportunities for health professionals wishing to pursue a clinical academic career. Fellowships to support the training and development of early-career clinical academics are now offered by a range of funders. The report *Developing the Best Research Professionals* (UKCRC, 2007) led to the establishment of a national Clinical Academic Training (CAT) programme. By promoting a partnership between universities and healthcare providers, in England support for clinical academic careers is now starting to become established, and government-funded training to gain recognised qualifications, such as a Masters degree or a PhD, has recently become available. The NIHR/HEE now fund a clinical academic pathway, which provides a range of academic opportunities, from internships through post-graduate and post-doctoral education to professorships. A fundamental priority of this programme is the 'integrated' approach that emphasises both clinical and academic input into creating new collaborative posts between a hospital NHS Trust and an academic institution (Health Education England, 2014). Information on the current NIHR programmes is available at: www.nihr.ac.uk/funding-and-support/funding-for-training-and-career-development/training-programmes/nihr-hee-ica-programme/.

Opportunities have also been developed in Scotland (NHS Education for Scotland, 2010) and Ireland (Department of Health and Children, 2003).

A key recommendation from the *Shape of Caring* report (HEE, 2015) was the development of Doctoral Training Centres (DTCs), which support clinical registered nurses academically, and encourage an increase in active 'on-the-ground' research within a sound support structure while providing a clear academic pathway. It was also recommended that registered nurses who choose to complete a thesis or Quality Improvement Project as part of a post-qualification preceptorship programme could regard these as an initial stage of research training that could later enable them to apply to study for a postgraduate research degree (such as an Masters Degree or PhD), in an area that makes a direct difference to frontline patient care. In response, doctoral training schools, open to nurses, midwives and allied health professionals have begun to emerge across the UK.

Health Education England (HEE) has a statutory responsibility to promote research. The Health and Social Care Act 2012, HEE Directions 2013 and the Mandate from the Government to HEE require HEE to 'develop a more flexible workforce that is able to respond to the changing patterns of service and embraces research and innovation to enable it to adapt to the changing demands of public health, healthcare and care services (DH, 2014b: 29). HEE also has a statutory responsibility and mandate to undertake the development of a transparent and integrated multi-professional clinical academic career framework, which enables all partners to be clear about the strategic approach to developing the clinical academic workforce for patient benefit, and a specific objective to 'support clinical academic careers for health professionals and also seek to increase numbers of staff across all clinical and public health professions with a proper understanding of research and its role in improving health outcomes, including an ability to participate in and utilise the result of research' (DH, 2014b: 30). Indeed, integrated infrastructure across the health and educational sectors is key to the success and sustainability of clinical academic careers for individual practitioners, as they cannot happen in isolation. The national strategy for their development emphasises the role and importance of leadership in clinical teams so it is essential that clinical academics are equipped with the skills needed to examine the optimal characteristics of the workplace environment such that they can influence colleagues to foster the development of a research culture in their own clinical setting. This should include discussion of how to maximise input from those in different professional or clinical settings and how to influence others to adopt an inclusive approach across the wider clinical arena, incorporating multi-disciplinary staff.

Barriers to successful implementation of training programmes for clinical academics have been identified (such as the competing immediate and longer-term demands faced by managers in the clinical setting). In acknowledgement of this, a number of initiatives have been put in place to support managers in the support of others. For example, a recent toolkit for NHS managers to provide support for clinical practice in the development of clinical academic careers has been published by AUKUH (www.medschools.ac.uk/media/2325/aukuh-transforming-healthcare.pdf) as well as a handbook from NIHR, published as a negotiating prop through which aspiring clinical academics can begin difficult conversations (www.nihr.ac.uk/our-faculty/documents/Building-a-research-career-handbook.pdf).

It has been acknowledged (Willis Commission, 2012) that employers need to recognise the evidence regarding the benefits and return on investment of nursing, midwifery and allied health professional leaders who successfully combine practical clinical and academic work. Transforming the partnership between health and higher education requires a commitment to growing and developing clinical academic practice from within the current workforce.

Summary

- Educational programmes for registered nurses, midwives and allied health professionals are largely delivered at least at degree level or are moving towards doing so.
- There is increasing emphasis on the importance of content relating to research, including the generation, critique and implementation of evidence-based practice in pre-registration educational programmes.
- Opportunities for the development of clinical academic careers have been emerging for some years in the UK and elsewhere and are now becoming more readily available.
- The benefits of supporting health professionals to develop their research skills and experience while remaining as active clinicians has been established.
- Good collaborative working relationships between the health and educational sectors are crucial to the success of clinical academic career initiatives.

FURTHER READING

Clinical Research Network (2012) *Five-year Strategic Plan for Research Delivery 2012-2017.* London. NIHR.

Department of Health (2012) *Developing the Role of the Clinical Academic Researcher in Nursing, Midwifery and the Allied Health Professions.* London: Department of Health.

Medical Research Council (2015) *A Cross-Funder Review of Early-Career Clinical Academics: Enablers and Barriers to Progression.* A Review led by the Medical Research Council in collaboration with the Academy of Medical Sciences, British Heart Foundation, Cancer Research UK, National Institute for Health Research and Wellcome Trust.

National Institute for Health Research HEE/NIHR, *Integrated Clinical Academic Programme: For Non-medical Healthcare Professionals* (www.nihr.ac.uk/funding-and-support/documents/ICA/NIHR%20ICA%20Guide.pdf)

United Kingdom Clinical Research Collaboration (2007) *Clinical Academic Careers for Nurses, Midwives and Allied Health Professionals.* London: UKCRC.

United Kingdom Clinical Research Collaboration Subcommittee for Nurses in Clinical Research (Workforce) (2007) *Developing the Best Research Professionals Qualified Graduate Nurses: Recommendations for Preparing and Supporting Clinical Academic Nurses of the Future: The 'Finch' Report.* London: UKCRC.

USEFUL WEBLINKS

Academic Science Health Networks (AHSN): a network of 15 Academic Health Science Networks (AHSNs) was established by NHS England in 2013 to spread innovation – improving health and generating economic growth. Each AHSN works across a distinct geography serving a different population in each region. www.ahsnnetwork.com

The Association of UK University Hospitals (AUKUH) is the key leadership body across the UK promoting the tripartite interests of university hospitals: service, teaching and research. Its role is to represent University Hospital Trusts' unique interests in partnership with other national bodies.

Collaborations for Leadership in Applied Health Research and Care (CLAHRCs) are funded by the National Institute for Health Research and undertake high-quality applied health research focused on the needs of patients and support the translation of research evidence into practice with the wider NHS and Public Health. They are collaborative partnerships between a university and the surrounding NHS organisations, focused on improving patient outcomes through the conduct and application of applied health research. www.clahrcprojects.co.uk

The Health & Care Professions Council (HCPC): the independent regulating body for health, psychological and social work professionals in the UK. www.hcpc-uk.org

The National Institute of Health Research (NIHR): funds health research and aims to ensure that the NHS is able to support the research of other funders to encourage broader investment in, and economic growth from, health research. Specifically the NIHR funds clinical academic training pathways. See: www.nihr.ac.uk/funding-and-support/funding-for-training-and-career-development/training-programmes/nihr-hee-ica-programme

The UK Clinical Research Collaboration (UKCRC): a forum which promotes a strategic approach to the identification of opportunities and obstacles to clinical research and aims to establish a network to enable people to work together to transform the clinical research environment in the UK. www.ukcrc.org

Conclusion to Part III

The aim of this section was to provide you with the necessary skills, knowledge and tools to enable you to make changes to your practice as appropriate and ensure your practice continues to be evidence-based throughout your career. Hopefully you have now:

- identified ways in which changes can be made to practice and issues you need to consider before making changes;
- considered how best to reflect on your experiences and used that reflection to enhance your practice;
- identified your needs in relation to lifelong learning;
- developed confidence in your ability to used evidence appropriately in the delivery of care.

This part ends with a crossword puzzle, with clues to words relevant to Chapters 10 and 11. The answers can be found on p. 224.

ACROSS

4. Theory said to underpin practice (8)
8. Learning aimed at ensuring knowledge/skills are up to date (8)
9. A form of analysis that allows you to identify areas for personal development (4)
10. Zone where people prefer to practise (7)

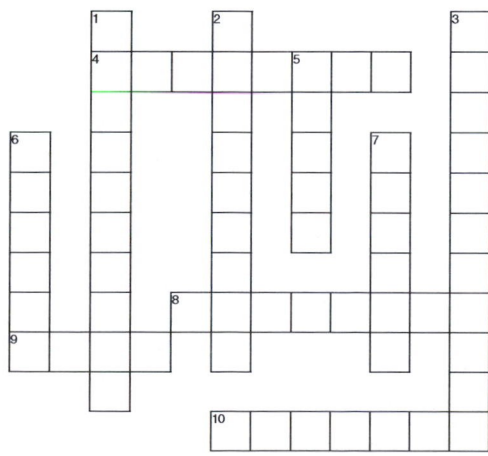

DOWN

1. Active appraisal of actions in a structured and critical way (10)
2. A collection of evidence demonstrating learning and development (9)
3. Someone who facilitates change in practice (11)
5. Framework for defining goals (5)
6. RCN framework for considering implementation of change (6)
7. Plan identifying how needs are met (6)

Appendices

Appendix 1
SWOT Analysis

Strengths	**Weaknesses**
What are my strengths? *What am I good at?*	*What are my current limitations?* *What might I do/think that would stop* *me meeting my goal?*
Opportunities	**Threats**
What will help in achieving my goal? *What resources are available to me?*	*What barriers are there to me achieving* *my goal – personal and organisational?*

Appendix 2
Template for Decision Aid

Date prepared ………………………………….

Name of intervention	
Aim of decision aid	
Description: *(mode of delivery, frequency, restriction)*	
How does it work?	
Extent of effectiveness	
Goal to be achieved	
What will be required of the patient?	
Benefits	
Risks	
Side effects	
Effect on quality of life	
Sources of further information	
References	
Other options *(it may be necessary to prepare individual sheets for each option)*	

Appendix 3

Formulating a Question and Searching for Evidence

1. Define your topic

What is your area of interest?

Break down your topic into key concepts using the PICO formula to create a clear clinical question:

Patient/problem	Intervention	Comparison	Outcome(s)

What is your question?

2. Define your scope/limits

Date range:

Language:

Type of studies:

Other:

3. Identify relevant resources to search

Appropriate databases to search:

4. Identify search terms

Consider any alternative terms/spellings, abbreviations, acronyms, etc. for your PICO concepts and list below:

Patient/problem	Intervention	Comparison	Outcome(s)

Check your selected databases for appropriate subject headings and include them in the table above. This information can then be used to build your **search strategy**. You can combine search terms together by using the Boolean operators '*and*', '*or*' and '*not*'.

5. Undertake your search and evaluate the results

Reflection on this learning experience:

Action(s) to be taken:

Appendix 4
General Critical Appraisal Tool for Research Studies

Section	Things to consider
Title	• Does it clearly identify the area of study?
Abstract	• Does it contain enough information for you to decide whether or not the paper is of interest to you?
Authors' qualifications	• Are these appropriate for the area of study?
Introduction	• Does it clearly outline the area of interest and give a rationale for the paper? • Is the research question and/or hypothesis clearly identified? • Is a theoretical/conceptual framework identified?
Literature review	• Is there a critical review of the literature related to the area of study? • Is the literature appropriate, up to date, mainly from primary sources, and does it include any seminal works associated with the topic?
Conceptual/ theoretical framework	• Are concepts clearly defined? • Is there a fit between the conceptual framework and the research design?
Ethical issues	• Has ethical approval been acquired? • Are the potential risks and benefits discussed? • Are sources of funding and outside interests identified?
Design	• Is the design clearly stated/described allowing for replication? • Is it appropriate to the study? • Are the strengths and limitations debated?

(Continued)

(Continued)

Section	Things to consider
Methodology	• Is this appropriate to the research question/hypothesis and aims of the study? • How are the data to be collected? • What sampling methods are used and are these appropriate to the methodology? • Are issues of reliability, validity, trustworthiness and rigour considered?
Results	• Does it give a clear description of how the results were reached? • Are the results clearly described and presented in a way that promotes understanding?
Discussion	• Are all the results explored and explained? • Is there consistency between the results and the arguments put forward? • Are the arguments logically developed and do they take account of opposing views? • Is the interpretation offered reasonable and does it make sense in light of what you know about the subject area?
Conclusions	• Are these logical and coherent? • Do these 'fit' with the data and the arguments presented in the discussion?
Recommendations/ limitations	• Are these presented in a clear way? • Is there a logical link between the findings and the recommendation?
Applicability to practice	• Is the sample used similar to the patients/service users in your area of practice? • Is training required to implement the findings? • Are considerations such as costs accounted for? • Do the benefits of changing practice outweigh any identified harmful effects?

Appendix 5

Summary Table of Study Details

Study details (full reference)	Pre-appraised evidence (Yes/No level 1–6)*	Study design (methodology and method)	Intervention/ phenomenon of interest	Setting (e.g. hosp/ community), geographical location, e.g. UK	Participants/ subjects (number, age, gender, ethnicity, cultural context)	Type of data analysis	Key findings	Quality	Applicability to practice

*Pre-appraised data hierarchy (DiCenso et al., 2009):

1. Systems
2. Summaries
3. Synopses of syntheses
4. Syntheses
5. Synopses of single studies
6. Critically appraised individual studies

Appendix 6

Critical Appraisal Tool for Quantitative Research Studies

Area	Issues for consideration
Hypotheses/research questions	• Are the research questions and/or hypotheses clear, unambiguous and where appropriate capable of being tested? • Are these consistent with the conceptual framework and research design?
Literature review	• Is there a critical review of the literature related to the area of study? • Is the literature appropriate, up to date, mainly from primary sources, and including any seminal works associated with the topic?
Conceptual/ theoretical framework	• Are the concepts clearly defined? • Is there a fit between the conceptual framework and the research design?
Operational definitions	• Are all terms used clearly defined? • Does it identify how variables will be observed and measured?
Design	• Is the design clearly stated/described allowing for replication? • Is it appropriate to the study? • Are issues which may result in bias minimised? • Are the strengths and limitations debated?
Data collection methods	• Are these adequately described? • Are the instruments adequately described and appropriate to the study's purpose and design? • Are the instruments used valid, reliable and reproducible?

Area	Issues for consideration
Sampling method	• Is the population of interest identified? • Are the subject characteristics clearly identified? • Are the inclusion and exclusion criteria clearly identified and appropriate? • Is the sampling approach appropriate to the design? • Is the size of sample identified and adequate? • Are power calculations present where appropriate?
Ethical issues	• Has ethical approval been acquired? • Are the potential risks and benefits discussed? • Are sources of funding and outside interests identified?
Data analysis	• Is it appropriate to the type of data? • Is complete information reported? • Is there adequate description of any subjects who were withdrawn from the study?
Findings	• Are these presented in a clear and understandable way? • Do tables/charts make sense? • Are data described in sufficient detail?
Discussion	• Is it balanced, including all major findings? • Are results considered in light of other research? • Does it address issues of generalisability? • Is there an acknowledgement of limitation?
Validity, reliability, applicability	• Are the results valid and reliable? • Is the relevance for practice identified?

Appendix 7

Critical Appraisal Tool for Qualitative Research Studies

Area	Issues for consideration
Research question and aims	• Is the question clearly stated and appropriate to the topic area? • Are the aims clearly stated and relevant to the research question?
Literature review	• Is there a critical review of the literature related to the area of study? • Is the literature appropriate, up to date, mainly from primary sources, and including any seminal works associated with the topic?
Conceptual/ theoretical framework	• Are concepts clearly defined? • Is there a fit between the conceptual framework and the research design?
Design	• Is the design clearly stated/described, allowing for replication? • Is it appropriate to the study? • Are the strengths and limitations debated?
Methodology	• Is a qualitative approach appropriate? • Is a specific approach used and described? • Does the research give a clear justification for the research design?
Reflexivity	• Does the researcher(s) provide a statement identifying their position/perspective?
Ethical issues	• Has ethical approval been acquired? • Are the potential risks and benefits discussed? • Are sources of funding and outside interests identified?

Area	Issues for consideration
Sampling/participants	• Is the sampling method appropriate and clearly described?
Data collection	• Are the data collection methods appropriate to the research approach and design? • Are the methods described in enough detail for you to understand the process?
Data analysis	• Is the data analysis tool identified and appropriate to the type of data and research design?
Findings	• Are the findings presented in a clear way? • Is there sufficient information to understand how the findings were reached? • Are the findings credible? • Are these discussed in light of other research/literature? • Are the study's limitations identified?
Conclusions	• Are these logical and coherent? • Do these 'fit' with the data presented and the arguments presented in the discussion?
Issues of rigour	• Have steps been taken to ensure the findings have **credibility**, transferability, **dependability, confirmability** and authenticity?
Applicability to practice	• Is the sample used similar to the patients/service users in your area of practice? • Is training required to implement the findings? • Are considerations such as costs accounted for? • Do the benefits of changing practice outweigh any identified harmful effects?

Appendix 8

Critical Appraisal Tool for Systematic Reviews

Area	Issues for consideration
Question	• Is there a clear and precisely defined question? • Are all terms/concepts clearly defined? • Are the inclusion and exclusion criteria clearly identified?
Search strategy	• What search terms were identified to search for studies, were these appropriate/exhaustive? • What databases were searched and were these appropriate? • Was a thorough search of all sources of literature undertaken, including grey literature?
Quality appraisal	• How was the quality of the studies assessed? • Is a checklist/tool identified for critical appraisal? • Did two or more reviewers appraise the literature? • Did the reviewers provide a rationale for exclusion of any studies?
Data extraction	• Has information about sample characteristics been extracted? • Is there sufficient information about the findings?
Summarising the evidence	• Where meta-analysis/synthesis is not used is this adequately justified? • Are the methods of 'pooling' data clearly explained? • Is the data analysis thorough and credible?
Meta-analysis	• Were two or more reviewers involved in the data extraction, ensuring the integrity of the data set? • Are treatment effects reported for all relevant outcomes? • How large is the treatment effect? • Is the heterogeneity of treatment effects adequately addressed?
Meta-synthesis	• Were two or more reviewers involved in the data extraction, ensuring the integrity of the data set? • Is a fuller understanding of the phenomenon of interest achieved? • Are the interpretations appropriate and sound? • Are examples of data provided to support interpretations?

Area	Issues for consideration
Conclusions	• Are these coherent and do they flow from the findings? • Is the strength of the evidence discussed?
Recommendations/ limitations	• What recommendations are made? • Are potential limitations identified?
Applicability to practice	• Are implications for practice explored? • How similar is the population of the studies to the patient group you are interested in?

Appendix 9
Action Planning

Goal: *What do I want to achieve?*
Rationale: *Why?*
Action: *How will I go about it?*
Criteria for success: *How will I know when I've got there?*
Evaluation: *What have I achieved and what next?*

Appendix 10
Personal Development Plan

What do I want to achieve? (goals)	How will this help my personal development?	How will I achieve it?	What help do I need?
1.			
2.			
3.			
Evaluation:			

Solutions to Word Puzzles

SOLUTION TO PART I CROSSWORD

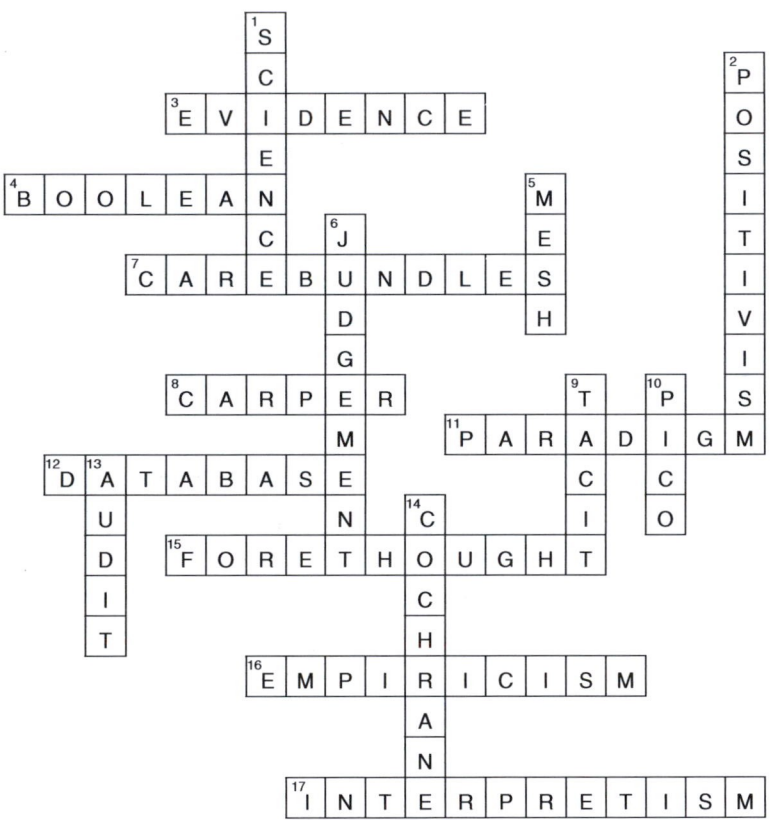

SOLUTION TO PART II WORD SEARCH

Hidden words:

VALIDITY; RELIABILITY; TRUSTWORTHINESS; CREDIBILITY; DEPEND-ABILITY; COMFIRMABILITY; TRANSFERABILITY; RIGOUR; VARIABLE; HYPOTHESIS; PROBABILITY; STRATIFIED; ETIC; EMIC; BRACKETING; METAANALYSIS; RANDOMISED; TRIAL; SNOWBALL; MEAN; MODE

J	T	R	I	A	L	U	O	U	T	Q	T	V	Q	U	X	T	E	V	X
A	G	M	U	Q	V	A	R	I	A	B	L	E	S	E	L	R	O	E	D
S	K	S	Q	Q	L	X	R	I	G	O	U	R	E	B	H	U	M	G	H
K	V	S	J	R	S	J	C	F	D	N	B	T	Y	T	N	S	N	Z	S
K	W	Y	B	F	N	K	O	Q	A	P	F	B	E	R	Z	T	J	R	T
M	A	Z	R	T	O	Q	N	N	Z	R	E	J	U	A	Z	W	D	A	R
O	V	H	A	T	W	E	F	Z	R	O	Z	F	I	N	Y	O	E	N	A
D	S	Y	C	D	B	Y	I	X	E	B	U	F	J	S	H	R	P	D	T
E	M	P	K	W	A	R	R	K	L	A	P	E	Q	F	F	T	E	O	I
R	E	O	E	A	L	E	M	E	I	B	T	T	L	E	F	H	N	M	F
Y	T	T	T	J	L	D	A	F	A	I	K	I	A	R	E	I	D	I	I
A	A	H	I	L	R	V	B	X	B	L	D	C	L	A	W	N	A	S	E
K	A	E	N	D	E	O	I	G	I	I	G	D	N	B	Z	E	B	E	D
E	N	S	G	I	Q	B	L	E	L	T	U	U	L	I	W	S	I	D	S
U	A	I	T	U	R	K	I	E	I	Y	F	G	K	L	Z	S	L	O	S
N	L	S	T	V	P	B	T	Z	T	F	F	Z	U	I	V	E	I	A	B
K	Y	C	W	R	W	J	Y	A	Y	M	E	A	N	T	K	R	T	C	P
L	S	U	J	E	M	I	C	B	A	S	N	K	M	Y	V	W	Y	G	O
S	I	U	F	R	T	Z	Y	P	R	I	V	A	L	I	D	I	T	Y	T
C	S	K	C	R	E	D	I	B	I	L	I	T	Y	T	D	F	R	C	B

SOLUTION TO PART III CROSSWORD

	¹R			²P					³C
	⁴E	S	P	O	U	⁵S	E	D	H
	F			R		M			A
⁶P	L			T		A	⁷A		N
A	E			F		R	C		G
R	C			O		T	T		E
I	T			L		I	I		A
H	I	⁸L	I	F	E	L	O	N	G
⁹S	W	O	T	O			N	E
	N						N
		¹⁰C	O	M	F	O	R	T

Glossary of Terms

Advanced decisions   recording of patient's preferences and care decisions in advance of care needs to ensure these are adhered to if ability or capacity to make decisions is impaired.

A priori   knowledge arrived at through reasoning processes.

Authority   knowledge coming from a source or person viewed as being authoritative.

Background question   generally a broad who, what, where, when, how, why question about an area of clinical interest.

Bracketing   a process used in qualitative research, where one's own thoughts and feelings in relation to the study are acknowledged and then 'placed on one side' to allow an unbiased analysis of the data.

Care bundles   three to five items of practice evidence grouped together in relation to a particular condition, treatment and/or procedure which have a more positive impact on treatment outcomes than any one single element.

Change agent   someone who facilitates change in the practice setting using specific interventions to implement and evaluate evidence-based practices.

Change management   the process of promoting change through the use of specific management theories and approaches.

Citation pearl growing   a way of identifying literature of interest by using an initial article (pearl) of interest to identify appropriate subject headings.

Clinical audit   an approach whereby clinical practices are measured against agreed explicit standards to promote clinical effectiveness.

Clinical effectiveness   the delivery of care in the most appropriate and evidence-based way.

Clinical governance   the process and structures put in place within healthcare institutions to promote and maintain quality of care.

Confirmability   the process of creating an audit trail of decisions taken in relation to analysis of qualitative data.

Correlation studies   quantitative research approach which examines relationships between variables without manipulation of the independent variable.

Credibility   processes put in place to ensure the findings of qualitative research are seen to be appropriate and representing the participants' experiences.

Critical appraisal   a careful evaluation of the worth, value or quality of evidence.

Cross-sectional studies   research which compares different groups within a population of interest, collecting data at a single identified point in time.

Data saturation   a term used in grounded theory research to indicate the point where no new information is being generated during the collection of data through the use of interviews.

Deductive reasoning   reasoning which moves from general theories to a specific hypothesis.

Dependability   a term used in assessing the quality of qualitative research, identifying the need to ensure all participant perspectives are accounted for in the analysis of data and presentation of findings.

Descriptive studies   quantitative research which observes, describes and documents areas of interest as they occur naturally.

Disproportional sampling   a form of sampling used in quantitative research where a larger sample of a particular subgroup (e.g. age, ethnicity) is used than is present within a population, usually where there is a need to consider the relationship between variables in that group.

Emic perspective   from the individual's rather than an outsider's or researcher's perspective.

Empiricism   a belief that only that which can be observed can be called fact or truth.

Etic perspective   outsider or researcher's perspective, rather than a research participant's perspective.

Evidence   an organised body of knowledge used to support or justify actions and beliefs.

Evidence-based medicine   an approach to the delivery of medical practice aimed at ensuring all activities are based on rigorous evidence.

Foreground question   a focused question formed in relation to a specific issue, looking for particular knowledge.

Grey literature   literature which has not been formally published, includes theses and/or dissertations, conference proceedings and in-house publications such as leaflets, newsletters and pamphlets.

Hermeneutics   related to meaning and interpretation – how people interpret their experiences within a specific context.

Hypothesis   a simple statement identifying a testable relationship between at least two clearly stated variables.

Inductive reasoning   reasoning which flows from thoughts related to a particular issue to a general theory.

Interpretivism   an alternative to positivism based on the belief that humans are actively involved in constructing their understanding of the world.

Intuitive knowledge   a form of tacit knowledge, which involves arriving at conclusions without being aware of thinking in a rational and logical way to generate that knowledge.

Lifelong learning   self-directed learning in which the aim is to ensure that knowledge and skills remain up to date.

Longitudinal studies   research in which data are collected at various points over an extended period of time from an identified individual/group of people.

MeSH terms   medical subject headings commonly used in certain databases to describe the contents of an article.

Meta-analysis   the pooling of data from a number of quantitative research studies to provide a larger data set.

Meta-synthesis   the pooling of findings from a number of qualitative research studies.

Non-propositional knowledge   personal knowledge linked to experience that is used by individuals to help them think and act.

Paradigm   a collection of ideas and concepts providing a theoretical perspective on how knowledge can be generated through research.

Participants   people who make up the sample in qualitative research.

Patient decision aids   tools generated through research and evaluation of patients' needs aimed at helping people make informed decisions about their healthcare treatment.

PICO question   format used to help to create a search question in relation to a particular clinical issue in which P = population; I = intervention; C = comparison; O = outcome.

Positivism   a belief that reality is ordered, regular, and can be studied objectively and quantified.

Proportional stratified sampling   a form of sampling used in quantitative research to ensure subgroups (e.g. by age, ethnicity) within a population are present in a sample in the same proportions.

Propositional knowledge   public knowledge, usually given a formal status by its inclusion in educational programmes.

Prospective studies   where data are collected in relation to a specific independent variable and the dependent variable is measured at a later date.

Publication bias   the tendency to publish studies that report positive results, resulting in a reported bias towards the effectiveness of a particular intervention.

Reflection   the process by which someone actively considers an experience, critically appraising it in light of experience and knowledge, and develops new perspectives to be tested in new situations.

Relevance   a consideration as to whether the findings from a study can be applied to the practice setting.

Reliability   concerned with identifying if the results of a research study are dependable and replicable.

Retrospective studies   research in which data are collected after an event of interest. For example patients' notes may be examined for information in relation to a specific treatment and recovery.

Rich (or thick) description   a term used in qualitative research meaning to give a full and thorough account of the research context, the meanings people attach to their experiences, their interpretation of issues and what motivates them to behave/respond in particular ways.

Rigour   ensuring that research is of high quality, conducted in an appropriate way, consistent with the underpinning philosophical principles.

Sampling units   people who form the sample within quantitative research, sometimes known as subjects.

Science   a body of knowledge, based on observation, experiment and measurement, organised in a systematic manner.

Search engine   an electronic device which enables you to search the World Wide Web for information.

Search strategy   A search strategy is the information (keywords, subject headings, etc.) that you enter into a database to find relevant evidence.

Secondary research research using data from primary research rather from an original source.

Service evaluation a systematic approach to gaining insight into patient satisfaction with services.

Shared decision making a partnership involving the sharing of information between at least two individuals (patient and health professional) to facilitate collaborative decision making.

Subjects people who form the sample within quantitative research, sometimes known as sampling units.

Systematic review a rigorous review of research findings in relation to a specific clinical question.

Tacit knowledge knowledge well known to practitioners but not evident within the research-based literature.

Tenacity a source of knowledge believed simply because it has always been held as the truth.

Transferability a term used in qualitative research to describe the tentative application of research findings from one study to another, similar group of participants.

Triangulation an approach used in qualitative research to increase the rigour of the findings. Entails considering the phenomenon of interest from different angles – usually in terms of its data, methodology, investigators, theoretical framework.

Trustworthiness whether data from a research study can be considered dependable and credible.

Validity whether or not the claims made in a research study are accurate.

Variables are factors or traits that are likely to vary from one person/situation to another such as weight, temperature, pain, personality traits.

References

Aas, R.W. and Alexanderson, K. (2011) 'Challenging evidence-based decision-making: A hypothetical case study about return to work', *Occupational Therapy International*, *19*: 28–44.

Adams, J.R., Drake, J.E. and Wolford, G.L. (2007) 'Shared decision-making preferences of people with severe mental illness', *Brief Reports Psychiatric Services*, *58*(9): 1219–21.

Akobeng, A.K. (2005) 'Understanding systematic reviews and meta-analysis', *Archives of Disease in Childhood*, *90*(8): 845–8.

Alper, B.S. and Haynes, R.B. (2016) 'EBHC pyramid 5.0 for accessing preappraised evidence and guidance', *Evidence Based Medicine*, *21*(4): 123–5.

Anfara, V.A. Jr and Mertz, N.T. (2006) 'Conclusion: Coming full circle', in V.A. Anfara, Jr and N.T. Mertz (eds) *Theoretical Frameworks in Qualitative Research*. Thousand Oaks, CA: Sage Publications. pp. 189–96.

Arnstein, S.R. (1969) 'A ladder of citizen participation', *Journal of the American Planning Association*, *35*(4): 216–24.

Association of UK University Hospitals (AUKUH) (2016) *Transforming Healthcare through Clinical Academic Roles in Nursing, Midwifery and Allied Health Professions: A Practical Resource for Healthcare Provider Organisations*. AUKUH Clinical Academic Roles Development Group.

Association of UK University Hospitals (AUKUH) (2017) National Clinical Academic Roles Development Group for Nurses, Midwives and Allied Health Professionals. AUKUH.

Barends, E., Rousseau, D.M. and Briner, R.B. (2014) *Evidence-based Management: The Basic Principles*. Amsterdam: Center for Evidence-Based Management.

Barker, J. and Linsley, P. (2016) 'Reflection, Portfolios and Evidence-based Practice', in J. Barker, P. Linsley and R. Kane (eds) *Evidence-based Practice for Nurses and Healthcare Professionals*. London: Sage. pp. 157–71.

Barr, O. and Sowney, M. (2007) 'Inclusive nursing care for people with intellectual disabilities using urology services', *International Journal of Urological Nursing*, *1*(3): 138–45.

Barredo, R.D.V. (2005) 'Reflection and evidence based practice in action: A case based application', *The Internet Journal of Allied Health Sciences and Practice*, *3*(3): 1–4.

Baston, J. (2008) 'Health decisions: A review of children's involvement', *Pediatric Nursing*, *20*(3): 24–6.

Batalden, P.B. and Davidoff, F. (2007) 'What is "quality improvement" and how can it transform healthcare?', *Qual Saf Health Care*, 16: 2–3.

Bengtsson J. (1995) 'What is reflection? On reflection in the teaching profession and teacher education', *Teachers and Teaching: Theory and Practice*, *1*(1): 23–32.

Benner, P. (1984) *From Novice to Expert: Excellence and Power in Clinical Nursing Practice*. Menlo Park: Addison Wesley.

Benner, P., Tanner, C. and Chelsea, C. (1996) *Expertise in Clinical Practice: Caring, Clinical Judgement and Ethics*. New York: Springer.

Best, D.E. and Hagen, S. (2010) *Shared Decision Making Interventions for People with Mental Health Conditions*. Chichester: The Cochrane Library/John Wiley and Sons.

Billay, D., Myrick, F., Luhanga, F. and Yonge, O. (2007) 'A pragmatic view of intuitive knowledge in nursing practice', *Nursing Forum*, *42*(3): 147–55.

BMJ (2007) 'Medical milestones, celebrating key advances since 1840', *BMJ*, 334(suppl): s1–22.

Boaz, A., Baeza, J. and Fraser, A. (2011) 'Effective implementation of research into practice: an overview of systematic reviews of the health literature', *BMC Res Notes*, 4: 212.

Boaz, A., Hanney, S., Jones, T., et al. (2015) 'Does the engagement of clinicians and organisations in research improve healthcare performance: A three-stage review', *BMJ Open*, 2015, 5: e009415.

Booth, A. (2004) 'Formulating answerable questions', in A. Booth and A. Brice (eds) *Evidence Based Practice for Information Professionals: A Handbook*. London: Facet.

Booth, A., Sutton, A. and Papaioannou, D. (2016) *Systematic Approaches to a Successful Literature Review* (2nd edn). London: SAGE.

Borton, T. (1970), 'Reach, Touch and Teach'. London: Hutchinson, Cited in Jasper, M. (2003), 'Beginning Reflective Practice Foundations in Nursing and Health Care', London: Nelson Thornes.

Boud, D., Keogh, R. and Walker, D. (1985) *Reflection: Turning Experience into Learning*. London: Kogan Page.

Bowling, A. (2014) *Research Methods in Health* (4th edn). New York: Open University Press.

Bradshaw, A. and Merriman, C. (2008) 'Nursing competence 10 years on: Fit for practice and purpose yet?', *Journal of Clinical Nursing*, 17(10): 1263–9.

Brady, N. and Lewin, L. (2007) 'Evidence-based nursing: Bridging the gap between research and practice', *Journal of Pediatric Health Care*, 21(1): 53–6.

Brown, R.A. (1992) *Portfolio Development and Profiling for Nurses*, Central Health Studies Series No. 3. Lancaster: Quay Publishers.

Bugers, J., Bailey, J., Klazinga, N., van der Bij, A., Grot, R. and Fender, G. (2002) 'Inside guidelines: Comparative analysis of recommendations and evidence in diabetes guidelines from 13 countries', *Diabetes Care*, 25(11): 1933–9.

Burnard, P. and Chapman, C.M. (1993) *Professional and Ethical Issues in Nursing: The Code of Professional Conduct* (3rd edn). Chichester: Scutari Press.

Butterworth, T., Jackson, C., Brown, L., Orme, M., Fergusson, J. and Hessey, E. (2004) StLaR HR Plan Project. Phase II Strategic Report. Developing and sustaining a world class workforce of educators and researchers in health and social care. A report to the Strategic Learning and Research Committee (StLaR) containing an account of present circumstances and suggested recommendations, leading to a Human Resource Plan for educators and researchers in health and social care. Project Report. Strategic Learning and Research Advisory Group (StLaR)/ National Health Service University.

Butz, A. (2007) 'Evidence-based practice in nursing: Bridging the gap between research and practice', *Journal of Pediatric Health Care*, 21: 53–6.

Caldwell, C. (2004) 'Practice development in child health nursing: A personal perspective', in B. McCormack (ed.) *Practice Development in Nursing*. London: Wiley.

Caldwell, K., Henshaw, L. and Taylor, G. (2005) 'Developing a framework for critiquing health research', *Journal of Health, Social and Environmental Issues*, 6(1): 45–54.

Canadian Nurses Association (2009) *Position Statement: Evidence-Informed Decision-Making and Nursing Practice*. Ottawa.

Care Quality Commission (2018) Experts by Experience. Available at: www.cqc.org.uk/about-us/experts-experience (accessed 27 August 2018).

Carper, B. (1978) 'Fundamental patterns of knowing in nursing', *Advances in Nursing Science*, 1: 13–23.

Carroll, J. and Johnson, E. (1990) *Decision Research: A Field Guide*. Thousand Oaks, CA: Sage.

Chinn, P.L. and Kramer, M.K. (2018) *Knowledge Development in Nursing: Theory and Process* (10th edn). St Louis: Elsevier.

Clarke, B., James, C. and Kelly, J. (1996) 'Reflective practice: Reviewing the issues and refocusing the debate', *Int J Nurs Sud*. 33(2): 171–80.

Clinical Research Network (2012) *Five-year Strategic Plan for Research Delivery 2012–2017*. London: NIHR.

Cochrane, A. (1972) *Effectiveness and Efficiency: Random Reflections on the Health Service*. Abingdon: Burgess.

Cochrane A.L. (1979) '1931–1971: A critical review with particular reference to the medical profession' in *Medicines for the Year 2000*. London: Office of Health Economics. pp.1–11.

Cochrane Bias Methods Group (2018) Assessing Risk of Bias in Included Studies. Available at: https://methods.cochrane.org/bias/assessing-risk-bias-included-studies (accessed 24 August 2018).

Cochrane Community (2017) Cochrane's 'Logo Review' Gets an Update. Available at: https://community.cochrane.org/news/cochranes-logo-review-gets-update (accessed 22 August 2018).

Colaizzi, P.F. (1978) 'Psychological research as the phenomenologists view it', in R. Valle and M. King (eds) *Existential Phenomenological Alternative for Psychology*. Oxford: Oxford University Press.

Cooke, A., Smith, D. and Booth, A. (2012) 'Beyond PICO: The SPIDER tool for qualitative evidence synthesis', *Qualitative Health Research*, *22*(10): 1435–43.

Cormack, D., Gerrish, K. and Lathlean J. (eds) (2015) *The Research Process in Nursing* (3rd edn). Oxford: Wiley-Blackwell.

Coulter, A. and Collins, A. (2011) *Making Shared Decision-Making a Reality: No Decision About Me, Without Me*. London: The King's Fund.

Council for Training in Evidence-Based Behavioural Practice (2008) Definition and Competencies for Evidence-Based Behavioural Practice (EBBP). Available at: https://ebbp.org/home/council (accessed 27 August 2018).

Coyne, I., O'Mathuna, D.P., Gibson, F., Shields, L. and Sheaf, G. (2011) 'Interventions for promoting participation in shared decision-making for children with cancer (protocol)', *The Cochrane Library*, 2.

Craig, J.V. and Stevens, K.R. (2011) 'Evidence-based practice in health care: What is it and why do we need it?', in J.V. Craig and R.L. Smyth (eds) *The Evidence-Based Practice Manual for Nurses* (3rd edn). Edinburgh: Churchill Livingstone/Elsevier.

Crowley, P. (1989) 'Promoting pulmonary maturity', in I. Chalmers, M. Enkin and M.J.N.C. Keirse (eds) *Effective Care in Pregnancy and Childbirth*. Oxford: Oxford University Press. pp. 746–64.

Dale, A.E. (2005) 'Evidence-based practice: Compatibility with nursing', *Nursing Standard*, *19*(40): 48–53.

Davies, K. and Gray, M. (2016) 'The place of service-user expertise in evidence-based practice', *Journal of Social Work*, *17*(1): 3–20.

Davies, P. (2004) Is evidence-based government possible? Jerry Lee Lecture, 2004. Presented at the 4th Annual Campbell Collaboration Colloquium, Washington, DC, National School of Government (UK).

Dawson, D. and Endacott, R. (2011) 'Implementing quality initiatives using bundled approach', *Intensive Critical Care Nursing*, *27*: 117–20.

Deegan, P.E. and Drake, R.E. (2006) 'Shared decision making and medication management in the recovery process', *Psychiatric Services*, *57*(11): 1636–9.

Deeks, J.J., Higgins, J.P.T. and Altman, D.G. (eds) (2011) 'Chapter 9: Analysing data and undertaking meta-analyses', in J.P.T. Higgins and S. Green (eds) *Cochrane Handbook for Systematic Reviews of Interventions Version 5.1.0* (updated March 2011). Available at: www.handbook.cochrane.org (Accessed 24 August 2018).

Deming, W.E. (1986) *Out of the Crisis*. Cambridge, MA: MIT Centre for Advanced Engineering Study.

Densen, P. (2011) 'Challenges and opportunities facing medical education', *Transactions of the American Clinical and Climatological Association*, *122*: 48–58.

Denzin, N.K. (2017) *The Research Act: A theoretical introduction to sociological methods*. New York: Routledge.

Department of Health (DH) (1989) *Working for Patients*. White Paper. HM Government.

Department of Health (1993) *A Vision for the Future: The Nursing, Midwifery and Health Visiting Contribution to Health and Health Care*. HMSO, London.

Department of Health (DH) (1997) *The New NHS: Modern and Dependable*. London: HMSO.

Department of Health (DH) (1998) *A First Class Service: Quality in the New NHS*. London: HMSO.

Department of Health (DH) (1999) Health Service Circular – *Making a Difference to Nursing and Midwifery Pre-registration Education*, HSC 1999/219: 1–18.

Department of Health (DH) (2001) *Valuing People: A New Strategy for the 21st Century*. London: HMSO.

Department of Health (DH) (2003) *Building on the Best: Choice, Responsiveness and Equity in the NHS*. London: The Stationery Office.

Department of Health (DH) (2005) *Mental Capacity Act*. London: The Stationery Office.

Department of Health (DH) (2006a) *Modernising Nursing Careers: Setting the Direction*. Edinburgh: The Scottish Executive.

Department of Health (DH) (2006b) *Agenda for Change*. London: The Stationery Office.

Department of Health (DH) (2007a) *Report of the High Level Group on Clinical Effectiveness*. London: The Stationery Office.

Department of Health (DH) (2007b) *Valuing People Now*. London: The Stationery Office.

Department of Health (DH) (2008) *Healthcare for All: Report of the Independent Inquiry into Access to Healthcare for People with Learning Disabilities*. London: The Stationery Office.

Department of Health (DH) (2011) *Innovation, Health and Wealth: Accelerating Adoption and Diffusion in the NHS*. London: The Stationery Office.

Department of Health (DH) (2012) *Developing the Role of the Clinical Academic Researcher in Nursing, Midwifery and the Allied Health Professions*. London: The Stationery Office.

Department of Health (DH) (2013) *The NHS Constitution*. London: The Stationery Office.

Department of Health (DH) (2014a) *Personalised Health and Care 2020: A Framework for Action*. London: The Stationery Office.

Department of Health (DH) (2014b) *Delivering High Quality, Effective, Compassionate Care: Developing the Right People with the Right Skills and the Right Values. A Mandate from the Government to Health Education England: April 2014 to March 2015*. 1 May 2014. London: The Stationery Office.

Department of Health (2015) *No Voice Unheard, No Right Ignored – A Consultation for People with Learning Disabilities, Autism and Mental Health Conditions*. London: The Stationery Office.

Department of Health and Children (2003) *The Research Strategy for Nursing and Midwifery in Ireland: Final Report*. Dublin: Stationery Office.

Dewey, J. (1933) *How We Think: A Restatement of the Relation of Reflective Thinking to the Educative Process*. New York: D.C. Heath and Company.

DiCenso, A., Ciliska, D.K. and Guyatt, G. (2005) 'Introduction of evidence-based nursing', in A. DiCenso, G. Guyatt and D.K. Ciliska (eds) *Evidence-based Nursing: A Guide to Clinical Practice*. St Louis, MO: Elsevier. pp. 3–19.

DiCenso, A., Cullum, N. and Ciliska, D. (2008) 'Implementing evidence-based nursing: Some misconceptions', in N. Cullum, D. Ciliska, S. Marks and B. Haynes (eds) *Evidence-Based Nursing: An Introduction*. Oxford: Blackwell Publishing.

DiCenso, A., Bayley, L. and Haynes, R.B (2009) 'Accessing pre-appraised evidence: Fine-tuning the 5S model into a 6S model', *Evidence-based Nursing*, 12(4):99–101.

Domecq, J.P., Prutsky, G., Elraiyah, T., Wang, Z., Nabhan, M., Shippee, N. et al. (2014) 'Patient engagement in research: A systematic review', *BMC Health Services Research*, 14: 89.

Dowding, D. and Thompson, C. (2004) 'Using judgement to improve accuracy in decision-making', *Nursing Times*, 100(22): 42–44.

Drake, R.E., Deegan, P.E., Woltmann, E., Haslett, W., Drake, T. and Rapp, C.A. (2012) 'Comprehensive electronic decision support systems', *Psychiatric Services*, 61: 714–17.

EBSCO (2018) CINAHL Take Away Guide. Available at: http://support.ebsco.com/promotion/promo_resources/Files/Col1/CINAHL/CINAHL_Take_Away_Guide.pdf (accessed 4 July 2018).

EBSCO Help (2018) CINAHL Subject Headings: Frequently Asked Questions. Available at: https://help.ebsco.com/interfaces/CINAHL_MEDLINE_Databases/CINAHL/CINAHL_Subject_Headings_FAQs (accessed 4 July 2018).

Ellis, P. (2010) *Evidence-Based Practice in Nursing*. Exeter: Learning Matters.

Elwyn, G., Laitner, S., Coulter, A., Walker, E., Watson, P. and Thomson, R. (2010) 'Creating a patient decision support platform in the NHS: A potential strategy for implementing shared decision making', *BMJ*, *341*: c5146.

E.M., Goldratt (1990) 'Theory of Constraints'. North River Press.

Eraut, M. (2000) 'Non-formal learning and tacit knowledge in professional work', *British Journal of Educational Psychology*, *70*: 113–36.

Evans, D. and Pearson, A. (2001) 'Systematic reviews of qualitative research', *Clinical Effectiveness in Nursing*, *5*: 111–19.

Facione, P. and Gittens, C. A. (2013) *THINK Crtically*. London: Pearson.

Faulkner, A. and Kent, J. (2001) 'Innovation and regulation in human implant technologies: Developing comparative approaches', *Social Science and Medicine*, *53*: 895–913.

Ferguson, L.M. and Day, R.A. (2007) 'Challenges for new nurses in evidence-based practice', *Journal of Nurse Management*, *15*: 107–13.

Fineout-Overholt, E., Melnyk, B.M., Stillwell, S.B. and Williamson, K.M. (2010a) 'Critical appraisal of evidence: Part 1', *American Journal of Nursing*, *110*(7): 47–52.

Fineout-Overholt, E., Melnyk, B.M., Stillwell, S.B. and Williamson, K.M. (2010b) 'Critical appraisal of evidence: Part 2', *American Journal of Nursing*, *110*(9): 41–8.

Fineout-Overholt, E., Melnyk, B.M., Stillwell, S.B. and Williamson, K.M. (2010c) 'Critical appraisal of evidence: Part III', *American Journal of Nursing*, *110*(11): 43–51.

Finlayson, K. and Dixon, A. (2008) 'Qualitative meta-synthesis: A guide for the novice', *Nurse Researcher*, *15*(2): 59–71.

Fitzpatrick, J. (2007) 'Finding the research for evidence-based practice. Part Two – Selecting the evidence', *Nursing Times*, *103*(18): 32–3.

Follett, B. and Paulson-Ellis, M. (2001) A Review of Appraisal, Disciplinary and Reporting Arrangements for Senior NHS and University Staff with Academic and Clinical Duties. A Report to the Secretary of State for Education and Skills, by Professor Sir Brian Follett and Michael Paulson-Ellis. September 2001.

Foster, N., Barlas, P., Chesterton, L. and Wong, J. (2001) 'Critical appraisal topics (CATs)', *Physiotherapy*, *87*(4): 179–90.

Foucault, M. (1979) *The History of Sexuality, Vol. 1*. London: Penguin.

Franck, L.S., Oulton, K. and Bruce, E. (2012) 'Parental involvement in neonatal pain management: An empirical and conceptual update', *Journal of Nursing Scholarship*, *44*(1): 45–54.

French, P. (1999) 'The development of evidence-based nursing', *Journal of Advanced Nursing*, *29*(1): 72–8.

Fulford, K.W.M. (2008) 'Values-based practice: A new partner to evidence-based practice and a first for psychiatry?', *Mens Sana Monographs*, *6*: 10–21.

Fulford, K.W.M., Peile, E. and Carroll, H. (2012) *Essentials of Values Based Practice: Clinical Stories Linking Science with People*. Cambridge: Cambridge University Press.

Fulford, K.W.M. and Stanghellini, G. (2008) 'The third revolution: Philosophy into practice in twenty-first century psychiatry', *Dialogues in Philosophy, Mental and Neuro Sciences*, *1*: 5–14.

Gawande, A. (2003) *Complications: A Surgeon's Notes on an Imperfect Science*. New York: Picador.

Gerrish, K. (2000) 'Still fumbling along? A comparative study of the newly qualified nurse's perception of the transition from student to qualified nurse', *Journal of Advanced Nursing*, *32* (2): 474–80.

Gibbs G (1988) *Learning by Doing: A guide to teaching and learning methods*. Further Education Unit. Oxford Polytechnic: Oxford.

Glaser, B. and Strauss, A. (1967) *The Discovery of Grounded Theory*. Chicago: Aldine.

Glasziou, P. and Haynes, B. (2005) 'The path from research to improved health outcomes', *Evidence-Based Nursing*, *8*(2): 36–8.

Glen, S (2009) 'Nursing education – is it time to go back to the future?', *British Journal of Nursing*, *18*(8): 498–502.

Goldacre, B. (2011) 'Foreword', in I. Evans, H. Thornton, I. Chalmers and P. Glasziou *Testing Treatments: Better Research for Better Healthcare* (2nd edn). London: Pinter and Martin.

Goldratt, E. (1999) *Theory of Constraints*. Great Barrington, MA: North River Press.

Green, J. and Thorogood, N. (2018) *Qualitative Methods of Health Research* (4th edn). London: Sage.

Green, S., Higgins, J.P.T., Alderson, P., Clarke, M., Mulrow, C.D. and Oxman, A.D. (2011) 'Chapter 1: Introduction', in J.P.T. Higgins and S. Green. (eds) *Cochrane Handbook for Systematic Reviews of Interventions Version 5.1.0* (updated March 2011). Available at: www.handbook.cochrane.org (accessed 27 July 2018).

Greenhalgh, T. (2014) *How to Read a Paper: The Basics of Evidence-Based Medicine* (5th edn). Oxford: John Wiley & Sons/BMJ Books.

Griffith, R. and Tengnah, C. (2012) 'Assessing children's competency to consent to treatment', *British Journal of Community Nursing*, *17*(2): 87–90.

Grol, R. and Grimshaw, J. (2003) 'From best evidence to best practice: Effective implementation of change in patients' care', *The Lancet*, *362*: 1225–30.

Grol, R., Wensing, M., Eccles, M. and David, D. (eds) (2013) *Improving Patient Care: The Implementation of Change in Health Care* (2nd edn). London: Elsevier.

Gülmezoglu, A.M., Chandler, J., Shepperd, S. and Pantoja, T. (2013) 'Reviews of qualitative evidence: A new milestone for Cochrane (Editorial)', *Cochrane Database of Systematic Reviews*, (*11*). Available at: www.cochranelibrary.com/cdsr/doi/10.1002/14651858.ED000073/full (accessed 9 November 2018).

Guyatt, G.H., Oxman, A.D., Schuneman, H.J., Tugwell, P. and Knottnerus, A. (2011) 'GRADE guidelines: A new series of articles in the Journal of Clinical Epidemiology', *Journal of Epidemiology*, *64*: 380–2.

Haas, J.P. and Larson, E.L. (2008) 'Compliance with hand hygiene guidelines: Where are we in 2008?', *American Journal of Nursing*, *108*(8): 40–4.

Hammond, K.R. (2007) *Beyond Rationality: The Search for Wisdom in a Troubled Time*. New York: Oxford University Press.

Health Education England (2014) *Research and Innovation Strategy – Delivering a Flexible Workforce Receptive to Research and Innovation*. London: Department of Health.

Health Education England (HEE) (2015) *Raising the Bar: Shape of Caring: A Review of the Future Education and Training of Registered Nurses and Care Assistants*. Lord Willis, Independent Chair – Shape of Caring review.

Health Research Authority (HRA) (2009) *Defining Research*. London: NHS Health Research Authority.

Health Research Authority (HRA) (2018) *UK Policy Framework for Health and Social Care Research*. London: Health Research Authority.

Herbert, R., Jamtvedt, G., Hagen, K.B., Mead, J. and Chambers, I. (2012) *Practical Evidence-Based Physiotherapy* (2nd edn). Edinburgh: Elsevier Butterworth Heinemann.

Heslop, P., Blair, P., Fleming, P., Hoghton, M., Marriott, A. and Russ, L. (2013) *Confidential Inquiry into Premature Deaths of People with Learning Disabilities (CIPOLD)*. Bristol.

Higgins, G., Spencer, R. and Kane, R. (2010) 'A systematic review of the experiences and perceptions of the newly qualified nurse in the United Kingdom', *Nurse Education Today*, *30*(6): 499–508.

Higgins, J.P.T., Altman, D.G., Gøtzsche, P.C., Jüni, P., Moher, D., Oxman, A.D., Savović, J., Schulz, K.F., Weeks, L. and Sterne, J.A.C. (2011) 'The Cochrane Collaboration's tool for assessing risk of bias in randomised trials', *BMJ*, *343*: d5928.

Higgs, J. and Titchen, A. (eds) (2001) *Professional Practice in Health Education and the Creative Arts*. Oxford: Blackwell Science.

Hoffman, K., Dempsey, J., Levett-Jones, T., Noble, D., Hickey, N., Jeong, S., Hunter, S. and Norton, C. (2010) 'The design and implementation of an Interactive Computerised Decision Support Framework (ICDSF) as a strategy to improve nursing students' clinical reasoning skills', *Nurse Education Today*, *31*(6): 587–94.

Hojat, M., Veloski, J.J. and Gonnella, J.S. (2009) 'Measurement and correlates of physicians' lifelong learning', *Academic Medicine*, *84*(8): 1066–74.

Huntington, A.D. and Gilmour, J.A. (2001) 'Rethinking representations, rewriting nursing texts: Possibilities through feminism and Foucauldian thought', *Journal of Advanced Nursing*, *35*(6): 902–8.

Hyde, A. (2009) 'Reflective endeavours and evidence-based practice: Directions in health sciences theory and practice', *Reflective Practice: International and Multidisciplinary Perspectives*, *10*(1): 117–20. Special Issue: Reflective Learning: Challenging Ideas and Creating Possibilities.

Iles, V. and Sutherland, K. (2001) *Managing Change in the NHS. Organisational Change: A Review for Health Care Managers, Professionals and Researchers*. London: National Co-ordinating Centre for NHS Service Delivery and Organisation.

Ingersoll, G.L. (2000) 'Evidence-based nursing: What it is and what it isn't', *Nursing Outlook*, *48*: 151–2.

Institute for Healthcare Improvement (2012) What is a Bundle? Available at: www.ihi.org/knowledge/Pages/ImprovementStories/WhatIsaBundle.aspx (accessed 20 August 2018).

Institute for Healthcare Improvement (2015) Science of Improvement. Available at: www.ihi.org/about/pages/scienceofimprovement.aspx (accessed 20 August 2018).

Institute of Medicine (2001) *Crossing the Quality Chasm: A New Health System for the 21st Century*. Washington DC: National Academy Press.

Jarvis, I.L. (1972) *Victims of Groupthink: A Psychological Study of Foreign-policy Decisions and Fiascoes*. Boston: Houghton, Mifflin.

Jasper, M. (1996) 'The first year as a staff nurse: The experiences of a first cohort of Project 2000 nurses in a demonstration district', *Journal of Advanced Nursing*, *24*: 779–90.

Jennings, E.T. and Hall, J.L. (2011) 'Evidence-based practice and the use of information in state agency decision making', *Journal of Public Administration Research and Theory*, *22*(2): 245–66.

Jivanjee, P., Pendell, K., Nissen, L. and Goodluck, C. (2015) 'Lifelong learning in social work: A qualitative exploration with social work practitioners, students, and field instructors', *Advances in Social Work*, *16*(2): 260–75.

Joanna Briggs Institute (2014) *The Joanna Briggs Institute Reviewers' Manual: Methodology for JBI Mixed Methods Systematic Reviews*. Adelaide: Joanna Briggs Institute, University of Adelaide. Available at: http://joannabriggs.org/assets/docs/sumari/ReviewersManual_Mixed-Methods-Review-Methods-2014-ch1.pdf (accessed 17 August 2018).

Johns C (1995) 'Framing learning through reflection within Carper's fundamental ways of knowing in nursing'. *Journal of Advanced Nursing*. 22: 226–34.

Justice, L.M. (2010) 'When craft and science collide: Improving therapeutic practices through evidence-based innovations', *International Journal of Speech-Language Pathology*, *12*(2): 79–86.

Kerlinger, F.N. (1999) *Foundations of Behavioural Research* (4th edn). New York: Holt, Rinehart & Winston.

Khan, K., Kunz, R., Kleijnen, J. and Antes, G. (2011) *Systematic Reviews to Support Evidence-based Medicine: How to Review and Apply Findings of Healthcare Research* (2nd edn). Boca Raton, FL: CRC Press.

King, A. (1995) 'Designing the instructional process to enhance critical thinking across the curriculum: Inquiring minds really do want to know: Using questioning to teach critical thinking', *Teaching of Psychology*, *22*(1): 13–17.

Kitson, A. (1994) *Clinical Nursing Practice Development and Research Activity in the Oxford Region*. Oxford: National Institute for Nursing/Centre for Practice Development and Research.

Kitson, A. (2002) 'Recognising relationships: Reflections on evidence-based practice', *Nursing Inquiry*, *9*(3): 179–86.

Knowles, M. (1990) *The Adult Learner: A Neglected Species*. Houston, TX: Gulf Publishing Company.

Kolb, D. (1984) *Experiential Learning: Experience as the Sources of Learning and Development*. New York: Prentice Hall.

Kristensen, N., Nymann, C. and Konradsen, H. (2016) 'Implementing research results in clinical-practice – the experiences of healthcare professionals', *BMC Health Res.*, *16*: 48.

Kuhn, T. (1970) *The Structure of Scientific Revolution* (2nd edn). Chicago: University of Chicago Press.

Lachal, J., Revah-Levy, A., Orri, M. and Moro, M.R. (2017) Metasynthesis: An original method to synthesize qualitative literature in psychiatry. *Frontiers in Psychiatry*, *8*: 269. Available at: www.ncbi.nlm.nih.gov/pmc/articles/PMC5716974/ (accessed 17 August 2018).

Lamb, B. and Sevdalis, N. (2011) 'How do nurses make decisions?', *International Journal of Nursing Studies*, *48*: 281–4.

Lanfear, D.E., Jones, P.G., Cresci, S., Khan, K., Kunz, R., Kleijnen, J. and Antes, G. (2011) *Systematic Reviews to Support Evidence-based Medicine: How to Review and Apply Findings of Healthcare Research* (2nd edn). Boca Raton, FL: CRC Press.

Lansisalmi, H., Kivimaki, M., Aalto, P. and Ruoranen, R. (2006) 'Innovation in healthcare: A systematic review of recent research', *Nursing Science Quarterly*, *19*: 66–72.

Lasater, K. (2006) 'Clinical judgement development: Using simulation to create an assessment rubric', *Journal of Nurse Education*, *46*(11): 496–503.

Lasater K (2007) 'Clinical judgement development: Using simulation to create an assessment rubric', *Journal of Nurse Education*, 46(11), 496–503.

Lasater, K. (2011) 'Clinical judgement: The last frontier for evaluation', *Nurse Education in Practice*, *11*: 86–92.

Leininger, M.M. (1985) *Qualitative Research Methods in Nursing*. Orlando, FL: Grune and Stratton.

Levett-Jones, T., Hoffman, K., Dempsey, J., Jeoong, S.Y., Noble, D., Norton, C.A., Roche, J. and Hickey, N. (2010) 'The "five rights" of clinical reasoning: An educational model to enhance nursing students' ability to identify and manage clinically "at risk" patients', *Nurse Education Today*, *30*: 515–20.

Lewin, K. (1951) *Field Theory in Social Sciences*. New York: Harper Row.

Lincoln, Y. and Guba, E.G. (1985) *Naturalistic Inquiry*. Newbury Park, CA: Sage.

Linsley, P. (2006) *Violence and Aggression in the Workplace: A Practical Guide for All Healthcare Staff*. London: CRC Press.

LoBiondo-Wood, G. and Haber, J. (2017) *Nursing Research: Methods and Critical Appraisal for Evidence-based Practice*. St. Louis: Mosby Elsevier.

Löffler, E. (2009) 'A future research agenda for co-production: Overview paper', in Local Authorities & Research Councils' Initiative (2010) Co-production: A series of commissioned reports. Swindon: Research Councils UK.

Maben, J. and Macleod-Clark, J. (1998) 'Making the transition from student to staff nurse', *Nursing Times*, *92*(44): 28–31.

Maher, L. and Panny, J. (2005) 'Service improvement', in E. Peck (ed.) *Organisational Development in Healthcare: Approaches, Innovations and Achievement*. Oxford: Radcliffe Publishing.

Manley, K., Hardy, S., Titchen, A., Garbett, R. and McCormack, B. (2005) *Changing Patients' Worlds through Nursing Expertise*. London: RCN.

Manley, K., McCormack, B., Wilson, V. and Thoms, D. (2008) 'The future contribution of practice development in a changing healthcare context', in K. Manley, B. McCormack and V. Wilson (eds) *International Practice Development in Nursing and Healthcare*. Oxford: Blackwell.

Mantzoukas, S. (2007) 'A review of evidence-based practice, nursing research and reflection: Levelling the hierarchy', *Journal of Clinical Nursing*, 17: 214–23.

Mantzoukas, S. (2008) 'The research evidence published in high impact nursing journals between 2000 and 2006: A quantitative content analysis', *International Journal of Nursing Studies*, 46: 479–89.

Mason, T. and Whitehead, E. (2011) *Foundations of Nursing Theory* (2nd edn). Maidenhead: Open University Press.

McColgan, K. and Rice, C. (2012) 'An online training resource for clinical supervision', *Nursing Standard*, 26(24): 33–9.

McGonagle, I., Jackson, C. and Kane, R. (2015) 'The ten essential shared capabilities: Reflections on education in values based practice: A qualitative study', *Nurse Education Today*, 35(2): e24–e28.

McLaughlin, H. (2010) 'Keeping Service User Involvement in Research Honest', *The Bristish Journal of Social Work*, 40(5): 1591–608.

McLean, C. (2011) 'Change and transition: Navigating the journey', *British Journal of School Nursing*, 6(3): 141–5.

McMullan, M., Endacott, R., Gray, M.A., Jasper, M., Miller, C.M.L., Scoles, J. and Webb, C. (2003) 'Portfolios and assessment of competency: A review of literature', *Journal of Advanced Nursing*, 41(3): 283–94.

McSherry, R., Artley, A. and Holland, J. (2006) 'Research awareness: An important factor for evidence-based practice?', *Worldviews on Evidence-Based Nursing*, 3: 113–17.

Medical Research Council (2015) *A Cross-Funder Review of Early-Career Clinical Academics: Enablers and Barriers to Progression*. A Review led by the Medical Research Council in collaboration with the Academy of Medical Sciences, British Heart Foundation, Cancer Research UK, National Institute for Health Research and Wellcome Trust.

Melnyk, B.M. and Fineout-Overholt, E. (2018) *Evidence-Based Practice in Nursing and Healthcare: A Guide to Best Practice* (4th edn). Wolters Kluwer.

Mencap (2007) *Death by Indifference*. London: Mencap.

Metz, A.J.R., Blasé, K. and Bowie, L. (2007) 'Implementing evidence-based practices: Six drivers of success. Brief research-to-results', *Child Trends*, October.

Mi, M. and Riley-Doucet, C. (2016) 'Health professions students' lifelong learning orientation: Associations with information skills and self-efficacy', *Evidence Based Library and Information Practice*, 11(2): 121–35.

Michaels, C., McEwen, M.M. and McArthur, D.B. (2008) 'Saying no to professional recommendations: Client values, beliefs, and evidence-based practice', *Journal of the American Academy of Nurse Practitioners*, 20: 585–9.

Miller, C., Tomlinson, A. and Jones, M. (1994) *Researching Professional Education: Learning Styles and Facilitating Reflection*. London: English National Board.

Miller, S.A. and Forrest, J.J. (2001) 'Enhancing your practice decision making: PICO, learning how to ask good questions', *Journal of Evidence-Based Dental Practice*, 1: 136–41.

Moher, D., Liberati, A., Tetzlaff, J., Altman, D.G. and The PRISMA Group (2009) 'Preferred reporting items for systematic reviews and meta-analyses: The PRISMA Statement', *PLoS Medicine* 6(7): e1000097. Available at: http://journals.plos.org/plosmedicine/article?id=10.1371/journal.pmed.1000097 (accessed 24 August 2018).

Monaghan, T. (2015) 'A critical analysis of the literature and theoretical perspectives on theory-practice gap amongst newly qualified nurses within the United Kingdom', *Nurse Education Today*, 35(8): 1–7.

Moon, J (1999) *Reflection in Learning and Professional Development*. London: RoutledgeFalmer.

Moore, L. and Kirk, S. (2010) 'A literature review of children's and young people's participation in decisions relating to health care', *Journal of Clinical Nursing*, 19: 2215–25.

Moule, P. Aveyard, H. and Goodman, M. (2016) *Nursing Research: An Introduction* (3rd edn). London: Sage.

Muir Gray, J.A. (1997) *Evidence-based Health Care: How to Make Health Policy and Management Decisions*. London: Churchill Livingstone.

Mulhall, A. and Le May, A. (2001) *Taking Action: Moving towards Evidence-Based Practice*. London: The Foundation of Nursing Studies.

Mullhall, P.L. (1993) 'Unknowing: Towards another pattern of knowing', *Nursing Outlook, 41*: 125–8.

Nairn, S. (2012) 'A critical realists' approach to knowledge: Implications for evidence-based practice in and beyond nursing', *Nursing Inquiry, 19*(1): 6–17.

National Institute for Health and Clinical Excellence (NICE) (2009) *Schizophrenia: Care Interventions in the Treatment and Management of Schizophrenia in Adults in Primary and Secondary Care*, Clinical Guideline No. 82 (updated edn). London: NICE.

National Institute for Health and Clinical Excellence (NICE) (2011) *Service User Experience in Adult Mental Health. Improving the Experience of Care for People using Adult NHS Mental Health Services*, Clinical Guideline No. 136. London: NICE.

National Institute for Health and Clinical Excellence (NICE) (2018) *Shared Decision Making*. Available at: www.nice.org.uk/about/what-we-do/our-programmes/nice-guidance/nice-guidelines/shared-decision-making (accessed 23 July 2018).

National Institute for Health Research (NIHR) (2010) *Involving Users in the Research Process. A 'How to' Guide for Researchers*. London: NIHR.

National Occupational Standards (2013) SFHM63: *Work with People and Significant Others to Develop Services to Improve Their Mental Health*. London: Skills for Health.

NHS Education for Scotland (2010) *National Guidance for Clinical Academic Research Careers for Nursing, Midwifery and Allied Health Professions in Scotland*. Edinburgh: NHS Education for Scotland.

NHS England (2014) *Mapping the Market II: Commissioning Support Services*. London: NHS England.

NHS Executive (1996) *Promoting Clinical Effectiveness: A Framework for Action in and through the NHS*. Leeds: NHS Executive.

NHS Institute for Innovation and Improvement (2005) *Improvement Leaders' Guide: Managing the Human Dimensions of Change, Personal and Organisational Development*. Available at: www.institute.nhs.uk/improvementleadersguides.

NHS Scottish Executive (2006) National Quality Standards for Substance Misuse Services. Edinburgh: Scottish Executive.

Nickols, F., (2016) 'Six Factors Affecting Performance Alignment' *Performance Improvement, 55*(3): 6–9.

Nielsen, A., Stragnell, M.S. and Jester, P. (2007) 'Guide for reflection using the Clinical Judgement Model', *Journal of Nursing Education, 46*(11): 513–16.

Nieswiadomy, R.M. and Bailey C. (2017) *Foundations of Nursing Research* (7th edn). Cranbury, NJ: Pearson Education.

Nind, M. and Hewitt, D. (2006) *Access to Communication* (2nd edn). London: David Fulton.

Noblit, G. and Hare, R.D. (1988) *Meta-ethnography: Synthesizing Qualitative Studies*. Newbury Park, CA: Sage Publications.

Nowell, L.S., Norris, J.M., White, D.E. and Moules, N.J. (2017) 'Thematic analysis: Striving to meet the trustworthiness criteria', *International Journal of Qualitative Methods, 16*: 1–13.

Nursing and Midwifery Council (NMC) (2017) *Revalidation*. London: NMC.

Nursing and Midwifery Council (NMC) (2018a) *The Code: Professional Standards of Practice and Behaviour for Nurses, Midwives and Nursing Associates*. London: NMC.

Nursing and Midwifery Council (NMC) (2018b) *Future Nurse: Standards of Proficiency for Registered Nurses*. London: NMC.

O'Byrne, P. (2007) 'The advantages and disadvantages of mixing methods: An analysis of combining traditional and autoethnographic approaches', *Qual Health Res*, *17*: 1381–91.

Ochieng, B.M.N. (1999) 'Use of reflective practice in introducing change on the management of pain in a paediatric setting', *Journal of Nursing Management*, 7: 113–18.

O'Connor, A.M., Llewellyn-Thomas, H.A. and Flood, A.B. (2004) 'Modifying unwarranted variations in health care: Shared decision making using patient decision tools', *Health Affairs*, *63*: 1–10.

Offender Health Collaborative (2015) *Liaison and Diversion Manager and Practitioner Resources: Service User Involvement*. Manchester: NHS England.

Omachonu, V. K. and Einspruch, N.G. (2010) 'Innovation in health care delivery systems: A conceptual framework', *The Innovation Journal: The Public Sector Innovation Journal*, *51*(1): 1–20.

Ormston, R., Spencer, L., Barnard, K. and Snape, D. (2014) 'The foundations of qualitative research', in J. Ritchie, J. Lewis, C. McNaughton Nicholls and R. Ormston (eds) *Qualitative Research Practice: A Guide for Social Science Students and Researchers* (2nd edn). London: Sage. pp. 1–23.

Oxford English Dictionary (2018) *Oxford English Dictionary Online*. Available at: www.oed.com/ (accessed 20 August 2018).

Page, S. (2002) 'The role of practice development in modernizing the NHS', *Nursing Times*, (98): 11, 34.

Page, S. and Hammer, S. (2002) 'Practice development – time to realize the potential', *Practice Development in Health Care*, *1*(1): 2–17.

Page, S. and Meerabeau, L. (2000) 'Achieving change through reflective practice: Closing the loop', *Nurse Education Today*, *20*: 365–72.

Page, M.J., Shamseer, L. and Tricco, A.C. (2018) 'Registration of systematic reviews in PROSPERO: 30,000 records and counting', *Systematic Reviews*, 7: 32. Available at: https://systematicreviews journal.biomedcentral.com/articles/10.1186/s13643-018-0699-4 (accessed 17 August 2018).

Pape, T.M. (2003) 'Evidence-based nursing practice: To infinity and beyond', *The Journal of Continuing Education in Nursing*, *34*(4): 154–61.

Parahoo, K. (2014) *Nursing Research: Principles, Process and Issues* (3rd edn). Basingstoke: Palgrave Macmillan.

Parkes, J., Hyde, C., Deeks, J. and Milne, R. (2001) 'Teaching critical appraisal skills in healthcare settings', *Cochrane Database of Systematic Reviews*, 3.

Patterson, C. and Chapman, J. (2013) 'Enhancing skills of critical reflection to evidence learning in professional practice', *Physical Therapy in Sport*, *14*(3): 133–8.

Patterson, C.M. and Newman, J.P. (1993) 'Reflectivity and learning from aversive events: Toward a psychological mechanism for the syndromes of disinhibition', *Psychological Review*, *100*(4): 716–36.

Pearson, A. (2005) 'A broader view of evidence', *International Journal of Nursing Practice*, *11*(3): 93–4.

Pearson, A., Field, J. and Jordan, Z. (2007) *Evidence-Based Clinical Practice in Nursing and Health Care*. Oxford: Blackwell.

Pearson, A., White, H., Bath-Hextall, F., Salmond, S., Apostolo, J. and Kirkpatrick, P. (2015) 'A mixed-methods approach to systematic reviews', *International Journal of Evidence-Based Healthcare*, *13*(3): 121–31. Available at: https://journals.lww.com/ijebh/Fulltext/2015/09000/A_mixed_ methods_approach_to_systematic_reviews.3.aspx (accessed 22 August 2018).

Peile, E. (2004) 'Reflections from medical practice: Balancing evidence-based practice with practice-based evidence', in G. Thomas and R. Pring (eds) *Evidence-Based Practice in Education*. Maidenhead: Open University Press.

Penny, J. (2003) 'Discipline of improvement in health and social care', in NHS Institute for Innovation and Improvement (2005) *Improvement Leaders Guide: Improvement Knowledge and Skills*. London: NHS Institute for Innovation and Improvement.

Petrova, M., Dale, J. and Fulford, K.W.M. (2006) 'Values-based practice in primary care: Easing the tensions between individual values, ethical principles and best evidence', *Br J Gen Pract*, *56*(530): 703–9.

Petticrew, M. and Roberts, H. (2003) 'Evidence, hierarchies and typologies: Horses for courses', *Journal of Epidemiology and Community Health*, *57*: 527–9.

Petticrew, M. and Roberts, H. (2006) *Systematic Reviews in the Social Sciences: A Practical Guide*. Malden: Blackwell Publishing.

Polit, D.F. and Beck, C.T. (2018) *Essentials of Nursing Research: Appraising Evidence for Nursing Practice* (9th international edn). Philadelphia: Wolters Kluwer.

Pope, C., Mays, N. and Popay, J. (2007) *Synthesizing Qualitative and Quantitative Health Evidence: A Guide to Methods*. Maidenhead: Open University Press.

Porter, S. and O'Halloran, P. (2012) 'The use and limitation of realistic evaluation as a tool for evidence-based practice: A critical realist perspective', *Nursing Inquiry*, *19*(1): 18–28.

Portney, L. (2004) 'Evidence-based practice and clinical decision making: It's not just the research course anymore', *Journal of Physical Therapy Education*, *18*(3): 46–51.

Price, R. (2009) 'Diploma to degree 1976–1993', *Radiography*, (*15*) Supplement 1: e67–e71.

PRISMA (2015a) *Preferred Reporting Items for Systematic Reviews and Meta-Analyses (PRISMA)*. Available at www.prisma-statement.org/ (accessed 17 August 2018).

PRISMA (2015b) *PRISMA for Systematic Review Protocols (PRISMA-P)*. Available at www.prisma-statement.org/Extensions/Protocols.aspx (accessed 24 August 2018).

Richardson, W.S., Wilson, M.C., Nishikawa, J. and Hayward, R.S. (1995) 'The well-built clinical question: A key to evidence-based decisions', *ACP Journal Club*, *123*(2), A12–3.

Rishel, C.J. (2013) 'Professional development for oncology nurses: A commitment to lifelong learning', *Oncology Nursing Forum*, *40*(6), 537–9.

Rossi, P., Lipsey, M.W. and Freeman, H. (2004) *Evaluation: A Systematic Approach* (7th edn). Thousand Oaks, CA: Sage.

Royal College of Nursing (2007) *Helping Students Get the Best from their Clinical Placements*. London: RCN.

Royal College of Physicians (2013) *Personalizing Healthcare: The Role of Shared Decision Making and Support for Self-Management*, RCP Position Statement. London: Royal College of Physicians.

Rycroft-Malone, J. (2002) 'Getting evidence into practice: Ingredients for change', *Nursing Standard*, *16*(37): 38–43.

Rycroft-Malone, J. (2004) 'The PARIHS Framework – a framework for guiding the implementation of evidence-based practice', *Journal of Nursing Care Quality*, *19*(4): 297–304.

Rycroft-Malone, J., Seers, K., Titchen, A., Harvey, G., Kitson, A. and McCormack, B. (2004a) 'What counts as evidence in evidence-based practice?', *Journal of Advanced Nursing*, *47*(1): 81–90.

Rycroft-Malone, J., Harvey, G., Seers, K., Kitson, A., McCormack, B. and Titchen, A. (2004b) 'An exploration of the factors that influence the implementation of evidence into practice', *Journal of Clinical Nursing*, *13*(8): 913–24.

Rycroft-Malone, J., Fontenla, M., Seers, K. and Bick, D. (2009) 'Protocol-based care: The standardisation of decision-making?', *Journal of Clinical Nursing*, *18*: 1490–500.

Sackett, D.L., Rosenberg, W.M.C., Grey, J.A.M., Haynes, R.B. and Richardson, W.S. (1996) 'Evidence based medicine: What it is and what it isn't. It's about integrating individual clinical expertise and the best external evidence', *British Medical Journal*, *312*(7023): 71–2.

Sackett, D.L., Straus, S.E., Scott-Richardson, W., Rosenberg, W.M.C., Grey, J.A.M. and Haynes, R.B. (2000) *Evidence-based Medicine: How to Practice and Teach EBM*. London: Churchill Livingstone.

Saks, M. and Allsop, J. (2012) *Researching Health: Qualitative, Quantitative and Mixed Methods* (2nd edn). London: SAGE Publications.

Sandelowski, M. and Barroso, J. (2007) *Handbook for Synthesizing Qualitative Research*. New York: Springer.

Sanderlin, B.W. and Abdul Rahhim, N. (2007) 'Evidence-based medicine, Part 6: An introduction to critical appraisal of clinical practice guidelines', *Journal of the American Osteopathic Association*, *107*(8): 321–4.

Schön, D.A. (1983) *The Reflective Practitioner: How Professionals Think in Action*. New York: Basic Books

Schön, D.A. (1990) *Educating the Reflective Practitioner: Toward a New Design for Teaching and Learning in the Professions* (The Jossey-Bass Higher Education series). San Francisco: Jossey-Bass.

Schön, D.A. (1994) *The Reflective Practitioner: How Professionals Think in Action*. New York: Basic Books.

Schulz, K.F., Altman, D.G. and Moher, D., for the CONSORT Group (2010) 'CONSORT 2010 Statement: Updated guidelines for reporting parallel group randomised trials', *BMJ, 340*: c332.

Scott, K. and McSherry, R. (2008) 'Evidence-based nursing: Clarifying the concepts in nursing practice', *Journal of Clinical Nursing*, *18*: 1085–95.

Scottish Executive (2006) *National Quality Standards for Substance Misuse Services*. Edinburgh: Scottish Executive.

Sidani, S., Epstein, D. and Miranda, J. (2006) 'Eliciting patient treatment preference: A strategy to integrate evidence-based and patient-centred care', *Worldviews on Evidence-Based Nursing*, *3*(3): 116–23.

Sidley, G. (2012) 'Advanced decisions in secondary mental health services', *Nursing Standard*, *26*(21): 44–8.

Siminoff, L.A. (2012) 'Incorporating patient and family preferences into evidence-based medicine', *BMC Medical Informatics and Decision Making*, *13*(3): S6.

Simon, D., Schorr, G., Wirtz, M., Vodermaier, A., Caspari, C., Neuner, B. et al. (2006) 'Development and first validation of the shared decision-making questionnaire', *Patient Education and Counselling*, *63*: 319–27.

Standing, M. (2008) 'Clinical judgement and decision-making in nursing: Nine modes of practice in a revised cognitive continuum', *Journal of Advanced Nursing*, *62*(1): 124–34.

Standing, M. (2017) *Clinical Judgement and Decision Making in Nursing* (3rd edn) Transforming Nursing Practice Series. London: Sage.

Stevens, K.R. (2013) 'The impact of evidence-based practice in nursing and the next big ideas', *Online J Issues Nurs*, *18*(2): 4.

Stillwell, S.B., Fineout-Overholt, E., Melnyk, B.M. and Williamson, K.M. (2010) 'Asking the clinical question: A key step in evidence-based practice', *American Journal of Nursing*, *110*(3): 58–61.

Straus, S.E., Glasziou, P., Richardson, W.S. and Haynes, R.B. (2019) *Evidence-Based Medicine: How to Practice and Teach EBM* (5th edn). Edinburgh: Churchill Livingstone.

Straus, S.E. and McAlister, F.A. (2000) 'From EBM to EBL: Two steps forward or one step back?', *Medical Reference Services Quarterly*, *21*(3): 51–64.

Strauss, A. and Corbin, J.M. (1990) *Basics of Qualitative Research: Grounded Theory, Procedures and Techniques*. Thousand Oaks, CA: Sage.

Streubert, H.J. and Carpenter, D.R. (2010) *Qualitative Research in Nursing: Advancing the Humanistic Imperative* (5th edn). Philadelphia: Lippincott Williams and Wilkins.

Tanner, C.A. (2006) 'Thinking like a nurse: A research-based model of clinical judgement in nursing', *Journal of Nurse Education*, *45*(6): 204–11.

The Learning Disabilities Mortality Review Annual Report (2017) Healthcare Quality Improvement Partnership. Available at: www.hqip.org.uk/resource/the-learning-disabilities-mortality-review-annual-report-2017/#.W-rwXZP7SUl (accessed 13 November 2018).

Think Local Act Personal (2011) *Making it Real: Marking Progress towards Personalised, Community-based Support*. London: TLAP.

Thomas, G. (2004) 'Introduction: Evidence and practice', in G. Thomas and R. Pring (eds) *Evidence-Based Practice in Education: Conducting Educational Research*. Maidenhead: Open University Press.

Thompson, C. (2003) 'Clinical experience as evidence in evidence-based practice', *Journal of Advanced Nursing, 43*(3): 230–7.

Thompson, C. and Stapley, S. (2011) 'Do educational interventions improve nurses' clinical decision making and judgement? A systematic review', *International Journal of Nursing Studies, 48*: 881–93.

Thompson, C., Aitken, L., Doran, D. and Dowding, D. (2013) 'An agenda for clinical decision making and judgement in nursing research and education', *International Journal of Nursing Studies, 50*(2): 1720–26.

Thompson, C., Cullum, N. and McCaughan, D. (2004) 'Nurse, information use and clinical decision making – real world potential for evidence-based decisions in nursing', *Evidence Based Nursing, 7*: 68–72.

Thompson, C., McCaughan, D., Cullum, N., Sheldon, T., Thompson, D. and Mulhall, A. (2001) 'Research information in nurses' clinical decision making: What is useful?', *Journal of Advanced Nursing, 36*(3): 376–88.

Thompson, D.S., Moore, K.N. and Estabrooks, C.A. (2008) 'Increasing research use in nursing: Implications for clinical educators and managers', *Evidence Based Nursing, 11*: 35–9.

Thompson, J., Barber, R., Ward, P.R., Boote, J.D., Cooper, C.L. and Armitage, C.J. (2009) 'Health researchers' attitudes towards public involvement in health research', *Health Expectations, 12*: 209–20.

Tidd, J. and Bessant, J.K. (2017) *Managing Innovation: Integrating Technological, Market and Organizational Change* (5th edn). Chichester: John Wiley.

Timmins, F., McCabe, C. and McSherry, R. (2012) 'Research awareness: Managerial challenges for nurses in the Republic of Ireland', *Journal of Nursing Management, 20*: 224–35.

Tonin, F.S., Rotta, I. Mendes, A.M. and Pontarolo, R. (2017) 'Network meta-analysis: A technique to gather evidence from direct and indirect comparisons'. *Pharmacy Practice, 15*(1): 943.

United Kingdom Central Council for Nursing, Midwifery and Health Visiting (UKCC) (1986) *Project 2000: A New Preparation for Practice, United Kingdom Central Council for Nursing, Midwifery and Health Visiting.* London: UKCC.

United Kingdom Central Council for Nursing, Midwifery and Health Visiting (UKCC) (1999) *Fitness for Practice: The UKCC Commission for Nursing and Midwifery Education, United Kingdom Central Council for Nursing, Midwifery and Health Visiting.* London: UKCC.

United Kingdom Clinical Research Collaboration Subcommittee for Nurses in Clinical Research (Workforce) (2007) *Developing the Best Research Professionals. Qualified Graduate Nurses: Recommendations for Preparing and Supporting Clinical Academic Nurses of the Future. The 'Finch' Report.* London: UKCRC.

University of Waterloo (2015) *Group Decision Making.* Available at: https://uwaterloo.ca/centre-for-teaching-excellence/teaching-resources/teaching-tips/developing-assignments/group-work/group-decision-making (accessed 13 November 2018).

US National Library of Medicine (2018) MEDLINE®: Description of the database. Available at: www.nlm.nih.gov/bsd/medline.html (accessed 4 July 2018).

Van Graan, A.C. and Williams, M.J.S. (2017) 'A conceptual framework to facilitate clinical judgement in nursing: A methodological perspective', *Health Gesondheid, 22*: 275–90.

Watson, L. (2003) *Lifelong Learning in Australia.* Canberra: Department of Education, Science and Training.

Weiss, C.H. (1998) *Evaluation: Methods of Studying Programs and Policies* (2nd edn). Upper Saddle River: Prentice Hall.

West, M.A. (1990) 'The social psychology of innovation in groups', in M.A. West and J.L. Farr (eds) *Innovation and Creativity in Work: Psychological and Organisational Strategies.* Chichester: Wiley. pp. 309–34.

White, J. (1995) 'Patterns of knowing: Review, critique and update', *Advances in Nursing Science, 17*(4): 73–86.

Wildridge, V. and Bell, L. (2002) 'How CLIP became ECLIPSE: A mnemonic to assist in searching for health policy/management information', *Health Information & Libraries Journal, 19*(2): 113–15.

Wilkinson, J. Powell, A. and Davies, H. (2011) *Are Clinicians Engaged in Quality Improvement?* The Health Foundation, May 2011.

Willis Commission (2012) *Quality with Compassion: The Future of Nursing Education. Report of the Willis Commission on Nursing Education.* London: The Royal College of Nursing.

Windish, D. (2013) 'Searching for the right evidence: How to answer your clinical questions using the 6S hierarchy', *Evidence-Based Medicine, 18*(3): 93–7.

Woodbridge, K. and Fulford, K.W.M. (2004) *Whose Values: A Workbook for Values-based Practice in Mental Health Care.* London: Sainsbury Centre for Mental Health.

World Medical Association (2004) *Declaration of Helsinki. Ethical Principles for Medical Research Involving Human Subjects.* Available at: www.wma.net/policies-post/wma-declaration-of-helsinki-ethical-principles-for-medical-research-involving-human-subjects/

Wuest, J. (2011) 'Are we there yet? Positioning qualitative research differently', *Qual Health Res, 21*: 875–83.

Yadav, B.L. and Fealy, G.M. (2012) 'Irish psychiatric nurses' self-reported sources of knowledge for practice', *Journal of Psychiatric and Mental Health Nursing, 19*: 40–6.

Yin, R.K. (2018) *Case Study Research and Applications: Design and Methods* (6th edn). Thousand Oaks, CA: Sage.

Zellner, K., Boerst, C.J. and Tabb, W. (2007) 'Statistics used in current nursing research', *Journal of Nurse Education, 46*(2): 55–9.

Index

Made in the USA
Lexington, KY
08 June 2019